MW01012391

DEDICATION

This book is dedicated to my wife and family
whose unstinting support has enabled me to pursue
my interest in sunlight and health.

DISCLAIMER

The Healing Sun is intended to provide information on the beneficial effects of sunlight. The advice given on sunbathing in the following pages has been compiled to this end, but it is not intended as a substitute for medical advice. The author and publisher cannot accept any responsibility for ill-effects of exposure to ultraviolet light or any of the therapies described herein. Sunlight treatment should not be substituted for professional care.

Contents

ACKNOWLEDGEMENTS

The subject of sunlight and health requires a multi-disciplinary approach. Accordingly, the views of engineers, architects, designers and practitioners of traditional medicine were solicited to complement the available medical advice. I also sought the advice of my agent Caroline Davidson, of the Caroline Davidson Literary Agency, without whose enthusiasm and expertise this book would not have seen the light of day. Martin Weitz of Focus Productions, Bristol, also contributed greatly during the course of our discussions about radio and television documentaries on the sun and human health.

The ideas, and suggestions in the following pages represent the opinions of the author and not necessarily those of the experts who very kindly shared their views on various aspects of the subject matter. I am most grateful to: Alex Attewell, Curator of the Florence Nightingale Museum, Dr S.S. Bakhshi, Consultant in Communicable Diseases at Birmingham Area Health Authority; Dr John Cason, King's College Hospital, London; Dr Damien Downing, Nutrition Associates, York; Dr D.S. Grimes, Department of Medicine and Biochemistry, Royal Infirmary and Queens Park Hospital, Blackburn; Professor J.J. Harding, Nuffield Laboratory of Ophthalmology, Oxford University; the late Mr A.J. Howrie of the Osborne Partnership, Ledbury, Dr C.D.D. Hutter, City Hospital, Nottingham; Professor Kay-Tee Khaw, University of Cambridge School of Clinical Medicine, Addenbrooke's Hospital; Dr S.N.G. Lo, School of the Built Environment, University of Ulster; Professor Barbara Mawer of the University Department of Medicine, Manchester Royal Infirmary; John Palmer, Building Research Establishment, Watford; Dr Angela Schuh, Institute für Medizinische Balneologie und Klimatologie, Munich, and Chris Ramsden, Chris Dyke and Anne Greer at the Medical Design Research Unit, University of Central England.

In order to make the book more accessible, I have not formally referenced books and articles in the text. There is a bibliography which includes all of the relevant sources which I hope will be of value to those who wish to examine any of the subject matter in greater detail. I would like to extend my thanks to the researchers and authors whose work I have referred to whom I trust will accept a citation of their work in lieu of an acknowledgement. Apologies to anyone who I have omitted to mention and for any mistakes, which are entirely my own.

I wish particularly to thank the staff of the following libraries for their help and patience: Birmingham Central Library; Aston University Library; The Wellcome Institute for the History of Medicine and the Barnes Medical Library at the University of Birmingham; and Mrs Janice Mayhew, formerly librarian of the Lord Mayor Treloar Hospital, Alton, Hampshire. Thanks also to Thierry Bogliolo, Faye Hamm and their colleagues at the Findhorn Press for their support and forbearance, and to Sandra Kramer whose editorial input has made such an improvement to the text. I also owe a great debt to John Palmer whose detailed comments on the early draft of this book were invaluable in helping me to convert the original manuscript into a more readable form, and to Robert Arnott of the Department of Ancient History and Archaeology, the University of Birmingham who assisted greatly with the classical references. I would also like to convey my thanks to Caroline Tonson-Rye, assistant editor of *Medical History,* for her help with my article 'Sunlight Therapy and Solar Architecture' which formed the basis of Chapter 4 of this book.

A number of practitioners gave freely of help and advice. I am most grateful to Giovanni Maciocia, José Lacy and Charmian Wylde for their insights into Traditional Chinese Medicine, and to Jackie Becker for putting her knowledge of homeopathy and vaccination at my disposal on so many occasions. I am also most grateful to Alan Sanders, Jo and John Harford, Professor Yan Hai, Mr Li Ke Jing and the Reverend Lee Chak Yan, all of whom were kind enough to try and pass on their knowledge of Tai Chi, Qigong and Aikido to me over the years.

I would like to acknowledge many others who generously provided support and information including: Margaret Boniface; Jill Brown; Kenneth Cabral; Marianne Crisp; Chris Donnelley; Stephen Gorwitz; Chris Howrie; Gill Hughes; Peter Martin; Lorraine Mooney; Ray Munns and Tim Welch. During the preparation of this book Monsieur Maurice André of Leysin was most helpful in supplying details of the heliotherapy of Professor Auguste Rollier, and I would also like to thank Madame Chapuis-Rollier for permission to reproduce the photographs of Professor Rollier's work. I am most grateful to Pam Bochel for her typesetting skills, and to the editors of *Medical History, Here's Health* and the *International Journal of Ambient Energy* who very kindly gave permission for me to reproduce text.

I hope that I have traced sources of all of the text and pictures still under copyright. However, should there be any acknowledgement inadvertently overlooked or referenced incorrectly, the error will be rectified in subsequent editions by the Findhorn Press Ltd.

I would like to thank the following for their permission to reproduce selected copyright material:

AACR Publications, Philadelphia, for excerpts from *Cancer Research:* Apperley, F.L., 'The Relation of Solar Radiation to Cancer Mortality in North America,' 1941, 1, 191–195, and Studzinski, G.P., Moore, D.C., 'Sunlight – Can it Prevent as well as Cause Cancer?', 1995, September 15, 4014–4022

APHA Publications, Washington DC, for the excerpt from the *American Journal of Public Health:* Garland, C.F., Garland, F.C., and Gorham, E.D., 'Could Sunscreens Increase Melanoma Risk?' 1992, 82, 4, 614–615

Dover Publications Inc., New York, for *The Ten Books on Architecture* by Vitruvius

Edward Arnold for *Sunshine and Open-Air: Their Influence on Health with Special Reference to Alpine Climates* by L. E. Hill, 1925 and *Health and Environment* by L. E. Hill and J. Argyll Campbell, 1925.

HarperCollins for the extract from *Breaking The Bonds* by Dorothy Rowe, 1991

Her Majesty's Stationary Office, London, for the excerpt from *Resistance to Antibiotics and other Antimicrobial Agents,* the House of Lords, Science and Technology Committee 7th Report, 1998

Humana Press Inc., New Jersey for the tables from *Epidemiology of Cancer Risk and Vitamin D* by Garland, Garland and Goreham in *Vitamin D: Molecular Biology, Physiology, and Clinical Applications,* 1999, edited by Michael F. Holick

Dr Julian Kenyon for permission to quote from his book *21st Century Medicine,* Thorsons, Northampton, 1986

The Medical Society of London for the excerpt from: Gauvain, H. J., 'Planning a Hospital', The Annual Oration, Transactions of the Medical Society of London, , 61, May, 1938, 246–261

Pearson Education for the extract from *The Natural House* by Frank LLoyd Wright, Pitman, London, 1971

Penguin Books for excerpts from *Pliny The Elder: Natural History – A Selection,* (Trans. J F Healy) 1991, and *Herodotus: The Histories,* (Trans. A de Sélincourt) 1972

The Pharaoh Akhenaten's *Hymn to the Sun* reprinted by permission of The Peters Frazer and Dunlop Group Limited on behalf of Jaquetta Hawkes from her book *Man and the Sun,* published by The Cresset Press: © Jaquetta Hawkes 1962

The Royal Institute of British Architects for the excerpt from *The Joint Committee on The Orientation of Buildings,* 1933

Springer-Verlag Gmbh & Co. KG, for *The Influence of Occular Light Perception on Metabolism on Man and in Animal,* by Dr F. Hollwich, 1979

The extract from 'Some Observations on Hospital Dust with Special Reference to Light as a Hygienic Safeguard', by L. P. Garrod, which first appeared in the *British Medical Journal* on February 19th, 1944, 245–7, is reproduced by permission of the BMJ, as is the extract from 'An Address on the Treatment of Gunshot Wounds', by Sir Berkley Moynihan, which was published in the *British Medical Journal* on March 4th, 1916, 333–339. The extract from 'The Share of the Sun in the Prevention and Treatment of Tuberculosis' from the *British Medical Journal* of the 21st October, 1922, 741–745, and from 'Obituary, Sir Leonard Hill', *British Medical Journal,* April 5th, 1952, 767–768 are also reproduced by kind permission of the BMJ.

The extract from Hippocrates comes from *Regimen* reprinted by permission of the publishers and the Loeb Classical Library from Hippocrates: *Works of Hippocrates, Volume 4,* translated and edited by W.H.S. Jones and E.T. Withington, Cambridge Mass: Harvard University Press, 1923–1931

The extract from *Sunlight Could Save Your Life,* by Dr Z. R. Kime, 1980, is reproduced by permission of World Health Publications, Penryn California

Photographic Credits

The Florence Nightingale Museum, London

The Medical History Museum, Copenhagen University for the photographs of Dr Niels Finsen and Light Therapy at his clinic.

Paul Cave Publications, Southampton, for permission to reproduce photographs from 'The Lord Mayor Treloar Hospital and College', by G.S.E. Moynihan, 1988

Staatliche Museen zu Berlin – Preußischer Kulturbesitz. Ägyptisches Museum, photograph of the Pharaoh Akhenaten (Photo: Margarete Büsing) and of Imhotep (Photo: E Grantz)

INTRODUCTION

The Healing Sun explores the benefits of exposing your body to the sun, rather than the dangers. It has been written with the aim of restoring a little balance to the currently rather one-sided debate on sunlight and its effects on human health. You may be completely unaware, as I was when I began the research for this book, that in the right hands sunlight is a medicine. Throughout history it has been used to prevent and cure a wide range of diseases, and a few doctors still use its therapeutic properties to good effect. However, at the present time it is widely held amongst certain sections of the medical profession and the population at large that the damaging effects of sunlight on the skin far outweigh any benefits. Public health campaigns reinforce this message in an attempt to curb the annual increase in skin cancers. Any illusions about tanned skin being a sign of health or providing more than minimal protection to further exposure to the sun's rays seem to have been dispelled. So why read a book on the positive effects of sunlight and sunbathing?

To put it bluntly; your life could depend on it. Sunlight may cause skin cancer, but there is also evidence that it could prevent a number of very common and often fatal diseases: breast cancer; colon cancer; prostate cancer; ovarian cancer; heart disease; multiple sclerosis; and osteoporosis. When combined, the number of people who die from these conditions is far greater than the number of deaths from skin cancer; which is why the current bias against sunlight needs, in my opinion, to be redressed, and why I would advise you to read this book.

But before going any further, let me explain how I came to write *The Healing Sun*. Usually books of this kind are written by doctors of medicine, or medical journalists, and not doctors of engineering. However, my background is a little unusual in that for many years, while I was designing or evaluating what could broadly be called solar energy technologies of one form of another — solar collectors; equipment for use in spacecraft; and energy-efficient buildings — I was also studying complementary medicine. Working alongside architects on one particular project I became aware of a 'lost' tradition of designing sunlit buildings to prevent disease, rather than to save energy, and I became interested in the healing powers of sunlight. I began to study the history of sunlight therapy and found that the physicians who practised this ancient healing art, and the architects and engineers who supported them in their work, used sunlight very differently from the way many of us do today. As I am particularly fond of sunbathing, and only really feel fit and well when I have a tan, this came as something of a revelation. So, in the following pages I have attempted to summarize what was known about sunlight therapy in the past. In comparing this with some of the latest findings from medical research on sunlight and health I have, as you will see, come to some rather controversial conclusions. In order to understand them fully, I would strongly advise you to read the whole book rather than go straight to the final chapter.

The sun transmits energy in the form of electromagnetic waves: radio waves; microwaves; infrared radiation; visible light; ultraviolet radiation; and x-rays. Only a small amount of the sun's energy reaches us, as most of it is filtered out by the earth's atmosphere, so solar radiation at ground level is composed of visible light, and ultraviolet and infrared waves. Until the latter part of the 19th century it was thought that the 'heat' of the sun — what we now know to be the infrared rays — caused sunburn. Then scientists discovered that it is the ultraviolet component of sunlight which causes the skin to tan, and they began to use ultraviolet radiation on skin diseases. They then found that they could get better results with sunlight itself.

Attitudes towards the sun and its healing powers have changed quite markedly throughout history, because of scientific discoveries of this kind, or changes in fashion. Pale skin has been, and still is, considered desirable in countries with agricultural economies where the majority of the population work outdoors, and where a suntan is the mark of the labouring classes. Down the centuries, the well-to-do have done their best to keep the sun at bay. Society ladies used veils, parasols, wide-brimmed hats and even skin-whiteners to keep their complexions 'pale and interesting'. But in the developed world, where comparatively few people work outside, the opposite applies: tanned skin continues to be fashionable and a sign of prosperity for many people, despite public health campaigns advising against sunbathing. Tanning in order to follow the dictates of fashion has little to do with health. A 'vanity tan' has little in common with the forgotten art of sunbathing for health. By the same token, enjoyment and appreciation of sunlight is very different from the carefully considered use of the sun's rays to treat serious diseases.

Sunlight therapy has a habit of being discovered and then falling from favour, and when this happens it disappears almost without trace, sometimes for hundreds of years. It was very popular at the beginning of the 20th century, but has since seen a dramatic reversal in its fortunes with the result that a great deal of knowledge about the healing powers of sunlight has been ignored or forgotten. Did you know, for example, that sunlight kills bacteria and is quite capable of doing so even when it has passed through window glass? Also, were you aware that sunlit hospital wards have less bacteria in them than dark wards, and that patients recover faster in wards which admit the sun? Perhaps not, but as infections actually caught in hospital are now the fourth most common cause of death after heart disease, cancer and strokes, it is worth bearing in mind.

In fact, your forebears were probably better informed about the sun's healing properties than you are: people hold very different views on sunbathing depending on when they were alive and where they happen to live. Take, for example, a typical well-educated resident of Essen or any industrial city in Germany in the 1920s. Let us say he had served in the German army during the Great War, was wounded, and returned home having recovered from his injuries. Someone in these circumstances would have held sunlight in much higher regard than many of us do today. He would probably been aware of the scientific discoveries that had been made about light in the years immediately before the war: in 1903 the Nobel Prize for medicine was awarded to the Danish physician, Niels Finsen, in recognition of his success in treating tuberculosis of the skin with ultraviolet radiation. Then again, during the war military surgeons may have used sunlight to disinfect and heal his wounds at a sunlight therapy clinic in the Black Forest, or a similar institution in the Swiss Alps. Had he contracted tuberculosis on his return to Germany, sunlight therapy, or heliotherapy as it became known, might have been used to aid his recovery. The physicians who supervised the treatment of his wounds or tuberculosis would have paid very close attention to the way he responded to sunlight and, in particular, how well his skin tanned. In those days, the deeper the tan, the better the cure.

Sunbathing for health in this way required the services of skilled physicians who knew precisely the conditions most favourable for their patients: the best time of day to expose them to the sun; the best time of year; the correct temperature for sunbathing; what foods to give; how much exercise to allow in each case; which type of cloud cover would let enough of the sun's rays through to cause burning and so on. Then, as now, the overriding concern was to prevent burning; but it was the actual process of tanning which dictated the progress of the treatment and whether or not it was successful.

During the 1930s sunbathing was encouraged as a public health measure. Diseases such as tuberculosis and rickets were common in the industrial cities of Europe and North America at this time and it became accepted practice to expose anyone considered susceptible to either of them to sunlight. So the sun was used to prevent disease as well as cure it. Also, architects were introducing sunlight into buildings to prevent the spread of infection because, as we have already seen, it kills bacteria. They designed hospitals and clinics for sunlight therapy and even included special window glass so that patients could tan indoors during bad weather — ordinary window glass prevents tanning because it acts as a barrier to ultraviolet radiation.

In marked contrast to our German friend of the 1920s, someone living in Britain today would have a very different impression of sunlight and its effects on the human body. The received wisdom is that there is no such thing as a safe or healthy tan, and that a tan is a sign of damaged skin trying to protect itself from further injury. Children and adults are advised to protect themselves from the sun; particularly during periods of sunny weather during the spring and early summer. They are to avoid the sun between the hours of 11 am and 3 pm and protect themselves with T-shirts, hats and sunscreens. As you can see, there has been a complete reversal in thinking on the subject.

Reasons for the current antipathy towards the sun are not hard to find. After the Second World War, improvements in housing and nutrition led to a marked decrease in the incidence of the very diseases which sunlight had been used to treat. When antibacterial drugs such as penicillin and streptomycin became widely available in the 1950s medical practice changed out of all recognition. These new drugs offered the prospect of rapid cures for a wide range of infections, and so the hygienic and medicinal properties of sunlight were no longer considered to be as important as they had been. Sunlight therapy became unfashionable, and was soon relegated to the position of historical curiosity.

More recently there has been a great deal of emphasis on the harmful effects of sunlight. There is now a 'hole' in the ozone layer to worry about, as well as a year-on-year increase in the incidence of skin cancer. Sunlight is undoubtedly a powerful accelerator of skin ageing, and can trigger cancer in susceptible individuals but, paradoxically, it is essential to our health. The human body needs sunlight to manufacture vitamin D by synthesizing it in the skin. The optimal level of vitamin D for health is not known, and so the amount of sunlight exposure needed to perform this vital function is still very much open to question. What this means is that warnings about sunlight being essentially harmful need to be treated with caution. Sunlight may cause skin cancer but, as you will see in the following pages, there is evidence that the sunlight could be crucial in preventing a number of diseases that are associated with low levels of vitamin D. Also, relatively little importance has been attached to the influence of nutrition in the genesis of skin cancer. Yet the limited amount of research carried out on the subject shows that what you eat determines how your skin responds to sunlight. The proportion of fat in your diet, together with the vitamin and mineral content of your food, could decide how likely you are to sustain skin damage in the sun.

The medical literature on sunbathing is contradictory: one field of investigation highlights the benefits while another stresses the dangers. One of the more unfortunate developments in modern medicine is a trend towards specialization. In these circumstances it is difficult not to be unduly influenced by the views of experts in one field or another and miss the wider picture. It becomes much more difficult to see the wood for the trees or, rather, the sunlight through the trees. Indeed, to fully appreciate the beneficial effects of sunlight it is sometimes advantageous to put aside conventional medical thinking altogether and look to other traditions of healing. Sunlight, when used as a medicine, does not lend itself to the western reductionist method of analysis: trying to fathom its therapeutic effects at a molecular level, to the exclusion of all else, may not be the best way to unlock its secrets.

The physicians who used sunlight on war wounds and diseased bones and joints at the beginning of this century knew sunlight therapy worked but were at a loss to know why. Lacking a scientific theory with which to explain the effectiveness of the treatment they had to rely on a largely empirical approach. One consequence of this is that it has been easy for subsequent generations of doctors to ignore or dismiss their methods and their results, which is regrettable. There is much that they can teach us so, in addition to reviewing their work, I have briefly examined the ways in which the sun has been used to heal in cultures other than our own. This has entailed going back to the very early history of medicine and that of architecture too as, historically, there have often been close links between medicine and building design. The first physician known to history — an Egyptian of the 27th century BC called Imhotep — was also one of the world's most celebrated architects.

When sunlight has been valued as a medicine, architects have often produced buildings which admitted the sun's rays. But when sunlight is out of favour with doctors, as is the case at present, there is little incentive for architects to make provision for it in their buildings. There has been a tendency for therapeutic properties of sunlight to be held in much higher regard during periods when prevention was considered to be as important as cure. In these circumstances the demarcation between physician and architect was often much less marked than is the case today. In the past, architects were encouraged to have some knowledge of medicine.

15

During the last thirty years the hygienic and medicinal properties of sunlight have had little influence on the building professions. Where solar architecture has been adopted it has been for the purposes of energy conservation rather than health; even though it has long been recognised that getting sunlight into buildings has a favourable impact on the well-being of occupants. Sunlight penetration into buildings is now regarded as 'beneficial' or 'desirable' but this aspect of design still receives a relatively low priority. Indeed, the benefits of getting sunlight into buildings, other than psychological, would not be obvious to anyone reading the current literature on building design. As we now spend so much of our time indoors, I believe the advantages of living or working in a sunlit space need to be more widely studied and appreciated than is the case at present.

Sunlight therapy was a medicine of the pre-antibiotic era, when infectious diseases were commonplace and the only defence against them was a strong immune system. Since then, for about fifty years, tuberculosis, pneumonia, septicemia and a host of other potentially fatal illnesses have been kept under control by antibiotics. Unfortunately an increasing number of bacteria are becoming resistant to drugs and there are signs that the development of new antibiotics is falling behind the ability of organisms to adapt and acquire resistance. If matters do not improve, then therapies which increase our natural resistance to disease, some of which are described in the following pages, may receive rather more attention than they have in recent years. The emergence of resistant bacteria may also come to have an influence on building design.

By adopting some of the techniques described in this book it should be possible to make more of the benefits of sunbathing and minimise the risks. There are medical conditions which are made worse by exposure to sunlight, and some drugs, such as antihistamines, oral contraceptives, antidiabetic agents, tranquillizers, diuretics and a number of antibiotics, increase sensitivity to the sun. Anyone about to embark on a programme of sunbathing should check with their doctor if they are in any doubt about their health or any medicines which they are taking.

The human race evolved under the sun, and the sun's healing powers have been worshipped for thousands of years. The aim of this book is to show how sunlight was used to prevent and cure disease in the past, and how it can heal us and help us now and in the future. The sun-god Apollo was the Greek god of medicine and there are two inscriptions from his temple at Delphi that give, perhaps, the best advice on sunbathing to be found anywhere: *'All things in moderation....Know thyself.'*

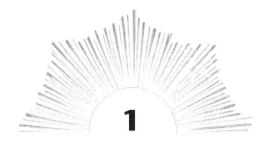

1

YOUR BODY AND MIND
IN THE SUN

Sunbathing is one of life's great pleasures. For some of us, exposing our skin to the gentle warmth of the sun's rays in the spring and early summer is, in a way, a form of sun-worship. We recognize that our bodies need direct contact with the life-giving sun as we emerge from the darkness of winter. The sun seems to strengthen us and lift our spirits. But why should this be so? Surely the sun has very little real influence over the physical and chemical processes of the human body? Many people seem to get along quite well with little or no sunlight and, of course, sunbathing causes skin cancer.

Well, until quite recently, relatively little was known about the effects of sunlight on human health. Although sunlight has been used as a medicine for thousands of years, no one really knew how or why it worked and they still don't. But during the last two decades, scientists have advanced their understanding of some of the more subtle physiological and biochemical responses of the body to the sun's rays and it is becoming clear that sunlight has a far more profound influence on our health than was once thought to be the case. Sunlight may cause skin cancer but, paradoxically, there is growing scientific evidence that the sun's rays could play a key role in preventing and ameliorating a number of serious degenerative and infectious diseases. These include cancer of the breast, colon, ovaries and prostate; diabetes; high blood pressure; heart disease; multiple sclerosis; osteoporosis; psoriasis; rickets and tuberculosis. Each of these conditions — and sunlight's influence on them — is examined in the pages that follow, but first let us see what sunlight does to the human body in broad terms.

Sunlight which reaches the earth's surface is made up of visible light, ultraviolet radiation and infra-red radiation. Approximately 37 per cent of the sun's radiation is in the form of visible light, 3 per cent is ultraviolet and the remaining 60 per cent is infra-red. The sun's rays contain two wavelengths that affect the skin: ultraviolet A, or UVA, (320–400 nm) and ultraviolet B, or UVB (290–320 nm). Both promote tanning and burning. UVB burns skin more rapidly than UVA, but does not penetrate as deeply. Until a few years ago UVA was thought to be relatively safe, but it is now known that these rays penetrate deeply into the skin. Chronic exposure to the sun for several hours each day, over many years, can cause permanent changes to the structure of the skin, leading to premature ageing. It can cause the skin to atrophy and, in susceptible individuals, cancers can develop. Acute episodes of sunbathing can also damage the skin, as anyone who has developed sunburn on the first day of their summer holiday will know to their cost. However, sunlight also has a beneficial effect on a number of common skin disorders, such as psoriasis, some forms of acne and eczema and a rare malignant skin cancer called *mycosis fungoides*. Sunlight has also been used to clear up bacterial and fungal infections of the skin. So the sun can heal the skin as well as harm it.

Vitamin D and 'The Vitamin D Winter'

Perhaps the most widely recognized benefit of exposing the skin to the sun's ultraviolet rays is that this activates the production of vitamin D, which is essential for the growth and maintenance of teeth and bones and a healthy immune system. Most of the world's population obtain all of their vitamin D from the sun and it is only people who spend long periods indoors who rely on their diet for this essential nutrient. By an accident of history, which will be discussed in due course, vitamin D is referred to as a vitamin when really it is a hormone. Vitamins are substances that cannot normally be synthesized in the body and have to be provided in the diet. Hormones are actually produced in the body and act as 'chemical messengers' controlling, amongst other things, growth, sexual maturation, reproduction and glucose levels in the blood. Only about a quarter of the vitamin D needed for this is available in a normal British diet, the rest should be produced by the photochemical action of the sun on our skin.

Although we are often told in popular books and magazine articles that relatively little sunlight is required for the synthesis of vitamin D and you only need to expose the face and arms for a few minutes to get your daily requirement, the seasonal nature of the process is not mentioned as often as it should be. In countries far from the equator such as Britain it is impossible to produce vitamin D in the skin from October to March. There is a very definite 'vitamin D winter' in this country and others at similar latitudes because UVB radiation with the right wavelengths to produce vitamin D in the skin is only present at ground level during the sixth months from April to September. The best months are May, June and July and even then most vitamin D is synthesized in the hours between mid-morning and mid-afternoon. During the winter months our vitamin D requirements are met from the store we build up during the previous summer's exposure to the sun. So, in other words, the skin has to be exposed to sunlight at regular intervals in the summer to get enough vitamin D to last through the winter.

When sunlight penetrates the skin it converts a prohormone, called 7-dehydrocholesterol, into pre-vitamin D_3. Then, over the course of two to three days pre-vitamin D_3 undergoes further changes in the skin to become vitamin D_3 which is then carried via bloodstream to the liver and then the kidneys to become the biologically active hormone 1,25 dihydroxyvitamin D_3. This is sometimes referred to as 'soltriol', which means 'hormone of sunlight'. Only about 15 per cent of the available 7-dehydrocholesterol in the skin actually becomes vitamin D_3, as prolonged exposure to the sun converts pre-vitamin D_3 into substances called lumisterol and tachysterol, which are both biologically inert. So prolonged exposure to the sun produces no more vitamin D than short exposures, which means that you don't have to tan for the process to take place. However, it is worth bearing in mind that the wavelengths that synthesize vitamin D in the skin are from 290–320 nm and the wavelengths that cause erythema, or sunburn, are 290–400nm, which means that if you block out the rays that cause burning you also prevent the synthesis of vitamin D.

Of course, if you limit your exposure to the sun's ultraviolet rays — by staying indoors or covering your skin with clothes and sunscreens — your reserves of vitamin D may be low for half of the year. This puts you at risk of developing a number of serious diseases related to vitamin D deficiency. You can avoid these problems by taking vitamin D supplements, but these are toxic at high levels and the body makes better use of vitamin D derived from the sun than it does from vitamin D in the diet.

The bones which form the human skeleton are made of living tissue, which changes all the time as new cells are added and old ones removed. Vitamin D maintains the correct balance of calcium and phosphorous necessary for this constant process of bone formation and remodelling. Most of the calcium in the body is stored in the skeleton with a small amount circulating in the bloodstream. Calcium is added and subtracted to and from blood and bone in a continuous process which can become less effective as we age. As we grow older our ability to utilize calcium can weaken and it then becomes increasingly difficult for calcium absorption to keep up with calcium loss. So bones tend to become thinner and weaker as bone mass declines. An additional factor in this process is that when vitamin D levels are low the body cannot absorb sufficient calcium to stay healthy, no matter how much calcium is taken in.

DEFICIENCY, OR INSUFFICIENCY?

Loss of calcium from the bones can be caused either by an insufficiency of vitamin D or by a deficiency. There is an insufficiency of vitamin D when the body tries to keep the amount of calcium in the blood at normal levels by increasing the amount of parathyroid hormone secreted into the bloodstream from the parathyroid glands. This, in turn, increases the amount of calcium being taken from the bones in an attempt to compensate for inadequate calcium absorption from the diet. Not surprisingly this condition, called secondary hyperparathyroidism, is known to be an important factor in age-related bone loss and can lead to an increased risk of fractures. But when vitamin D levels decline even further, deficiency — as opposed to insufficiency — occurs. The body can no longer maintain adequate levels of calcium in the bloodstream regardless of the amount of parathyroid hormone secreted and the skeleton loses calcium at an even faster rate.

Some experts regard secondary hyperparathyroidism as a pathological condition and recommend a minimum daily intake of vitamin D which will prevent insufficiency. Others base their recommendations on the amount required to prevent a deficiency disease. What this means is that there are no internationally agreed figures for the amount of vitamin D needed each day to stay healthy. As the optimal level of vitamin D for health is not known, the amount of sunlight exposure needed to maintain healthy bones is still very much open to question too.

In the United States the recommended daily allowance of vitamin D for adults up to 50 years of age is 200 IU (international units), increasing to 400 IU a day for those aged 51–70 years and 600 IU for those aged 71 and over, while in the UK the Department of Health has recently decided to stay with a figure of 400 IU for adults over 65, but no figure has been set from 4–64 years, as it is assumed that regular exposure to summer sunlight will ensure adequacy. A daily allowance of 400 IU is recommended for individuals in this age group who are particularly at risk of vitamin D deficiency, such as pregnant and lactating mothers. Significantly, the British diet supplies on average only about 100 IU, which is typical of many other developed countries. A diet that provided all of the daily requirement would have to include large amounts of fatty fish such as salmon, mackerel, herring and sardines and ingredients such as full-cream milk, butter, eggs, cheese and liver.

In the United States and some European countries milk and margarine are supplemented with synthetic forms of vitamin D, but these are not particularly reliable sources. The intake of these foodstuffs varies considerably from individual to individual and the amount of vitamin D contained in these products also varies. Studies have shown that less than 20 per cent of milk samples taken from across the United States contain the amount of vitamin D stated on the label. Vitamin D is added to foods as a public health measure to prevent rickets and reduce people's dependence on sunlight. The practice was widespread long before scientists had precise knowledge regarding the relative contributions of vitamin D from the sun and dietary vitamin D. It was only as recently as the 1970s that the status of vitamin D as a hormone, rather than a vitamin, was established and methods were developed for measuring the amount circulating in the bloodstream.

There have been calls for vitamin D to be removed from foodstuffs because of the risks of toxicity, particularly in children. A daily dose of about 2400 IU can cause hypercalcemia, or abnormally high levels of calcium in the blood, in adults. The symptoms include nausea, vomiting, excessive urination, extreme fatigue, depression and muscle weakness. Regular high doses of vitamin D can result in abnormal calcium deposits in blood vessel walls, the kidneys and other organs, coma and even death. The amount of vitamin D and calcium taken during pregnancy should be carefully monitored, as should the intake of lactating mothers. Vitamin D can trigger asthma in aspirin-sensitive patients and should be taken with caution by patients on anticoagulants. It can also cause a rise of blood glucose in insulin-dependent patients.

One of vitamin D's effects is that at the right levels it increases the absorption of magnesium from the diet. Magnesium is essential for a wide range of functions in the body, but one of the consequences of taking too much vitamin D is that the body excretes more magnesium than it would normally do and more is required to compensate for this loss. Excessive vitamin D intake causes magnesium deficiency in the heart, which can lead to spasm in the coronary arteries and, in extreme cases, a heart attack. It can also upset the body's calcium metabolism and may cause cholesterol levels in the blood to increase.

Happily, no one seems to have ever had a toxic dose of sunlight. Although human skin has the capacity to produce large amounts of vitamin D the process, as we have seen, is self-regulating. So, rather than relying on fortified foods or oral supplements, there is a great deal to be said for getting out in the sun for short periods during the spring and summer. The body actually makes much better use of vitamin D produced by the sun than the dietary form of the vitamin and if you get enough sunlight at the right time of year there is no need to have any dietary vitamin D at all. Alternatively, if you don't get out in the sun you could be vitamin D insufficient or deficient.

SUNLIGHT, CHOLESTEROL AND VITAMIN D

There are other consequences of limiting your exposure to summer sunlight besides vitamin D deficiency. We hear a lot these days about the dangers of high cholesterol levels in the blood but very little about the sun's role in lowering them. Cholesterol plays an important role in the body, being the precursor of the body's steroid hormones and similar in its molecular structure to vitamin D and to cortisone and the sex hormones we need for reproduction. At high levels cholesterol can cause damage to the lining of the arteries which can lead to high blood pressure, blockages and thromboses. What is not so well known is that sunlight can bring down blood cholesterol levels dramatically and that the human body actually needs ultraviolet radiation to break down cholesterol. Both the vitamin D precursor 7-dehydrocholesterol and cholesterol are derived from a substance called squalene. There is evidence that, whereas squalene in the skin is converted to vitamin D in the presence of sunlight, in the absence of sunlight it is converted into cholesterol. This would explain the high levels of cholesterol measured in populations at high latitudes and a seasonal variation of blood cholesterol which also has been reported: it seems cholesterol levels go up in winter, just as vitamin D levels fall and this is related to the amount of sunlight available.

Another striking effect of the sun's rays on the human body is on blood pressure. It has been known for more than half a century, from some of the earliest experiments with ultraviolet rays, that even a single exposure will lower blood pressure in normal individuals and can have an even more pronounced effect on individuals with high blood pressure. Research published in the *American Journal of Physiology* as long ago as 1935 showed that ultraviolet radiation reduced blood pressure in 60 to 70 per cent of hypertensive people. Some of the individuals who took part in these tests experienced falls in systolic pressure — the top number of the blood pressure ratio — of as much as 40mm/Hg. Diastolic readings — the lower figure — fell by 20mm/Hg in some cases.

If, as it appears, ultraviolet radiation can significantly reduce blood pressure, then it should come as no surprise to learn that blood pressure is generally highest in winter, when solar radiation is at its lowest levels, and lowest in summer when the sun's ultraviolet radiation is at its peak. Blood pressure is also affected by variations in skin pigmentation: greater skin pigmentation is associated with higher blood pressure. People of colour living in the United Kingdom and the United States have more hypertension than people of European origin. Conversely, when they are living in their indigenous regions — nearer the equator — they have lower mean blood pressure and lower frequency of hypertension and they rarely have the age-associated rise in blood pressure common to whites and African Americans.

Published data show a linear rise in blood pressure at increasing distances from the equator. They also show that geographic and seasonal changes in blood pressure are inversely associated with solar radiation. One explanation for the relationship between high blood pressure and low levels of sunlight is that if there is an increase in the production of parathyroid hormone, because only limited amounts of vitamin D are stored in the body, this may, in turn, adversely affect the structure and function of the vascular system. This hypothesis, which was proposed in the journal *Hypertension* in 1997, explains why dark-skinned populations living away from the equator are susceptible to developing hypertension, as they need significant amounts of sunlight to photosynthesize vitamin D.

The results of a study published in the *Lancet,* in 1998, showed that it is UVB radiation which lowers blood pressure, and that UVA radiation plays no part in it. So, theoretically, using a sunscreen which blocks out UVB radiation to prevent burning might also stop the synthesis of vitamin D, a reduction of cholesterol levels and a lowering of blood pressure. High blood pressure, or hypertension, affects an estimated 50 million people in the United States costing $2 billion dollars a year in lost earnings. The drugs prescribed to treat high blood pressure — a condition which is so common as to be considered almost a normal part of the ageing process in developed countries — are not without their side effects and the amount spent on medication for high blood pressure each year in these countries runs into billions. As hypertension is a risk factor for a number of serious conditions including stroke, heart disease and even cancer, their widespread use is understandable, but it seems that spending time outdoors in the sun offers a cheaper, if less convenient way of dealing with the problem.

Sunlight and Skin Type

Our earliest ancestors came originally from East Africa, one of the sunniest regions of the world. With the passage of time they gradually migrated north and south, well away from equatorial regions. The further they moved from the equator the lighter their skin became, which enabled them to form vitamin D efficiently during the relatively short summers at higher latitudes. This is probably something of an oversimplification but serves to illustrate the point that a suntan built up slowly is what many of us with pale skin were designed to have. Fair-skinned tribesmen and women would have worked outdoors for much of the year and would have tanned progressively. They would have gradually built up a good reserve of vitamin D during the summer in readiness for the winter. Their skin was well adapted to seasonal variations in the sun's ultraviolet rays. So is the skin of their descendants — but, unfortunately, we now spend so much of our time indoors that it has become difficult to tan safely, or synthesize vitamin D.

In strong sunlight a substance called melanin is produced in the skin and this forms the basis of a suntan. Melanin is a chemical compound which acts as a natural sunscreen and governs how much incident ultraviolet radiation reaches the deeper layers of the skin. Whether newly formed or already present in darker skin, melanin limits the amount of vitamin D produced. So, the more we tan, the more melanin is produced in the skin, with a corresponding decrease in vitamin D. This explains, in part, why it is impossible to get toxic levels of the vitamin from sunbathing. The other reason, as we have already seen, is that the synthesis of vitamin D in the skin is self-limiting; only a small proportion of the available prohormone in the skin becomes vitamin D_3.

Not surprisingly, there is a considerable difference between the amount of solar radiation needed to synthesize vitamin D in dark skin and in fair skin. Table 1 shows the amount of exposure each of the six skin types can withstand before burning. This gives a rough guide to the relative amounts of sunlight needed to synthesize vitamin D in each case. Some 20–30 per cent of UVB radiation is transmitted through the epidermis of white skin, but penetration is less than 5 per cent in deeply pigmented skin. So individuals with black skin require about six times more solar radiation to produce similar amounts of vitamin D than someone of Celtic extraction with Type 1 skin: enough to cause severe second degree burns in this most sensitive category. Anyone with very dark skin living at northerly latitudes could be considered at risk from vitamin D deficiency if they did not get prolonged exposure to the sun or take a supplement.

Table 1: Sunlight and skin type

Safe, healthy sunbathing requires moderation and a degree of self-knowledge, especially where the sensitivity of your skin is concerned. It is only by identifying your skin type, and paying close attention to how you tan, that you can work out how much exposure will be beneficial.

1 The most sensitive skin belongs to people of Celtic extraction: with red hair and blue or green eyes, or dark hair with green eyes. Typically their skin hardly tans at all and burns very easily, but with careful exposure they can increase their tolerance to sunlight. Someone with this type of skin who is unused to direct sunlight will burn after 20 minutes of British midsummer sunshine.

2 This is a very common skin type in people of northern European ancestry. Type 2s have pale skin, blond or red hair, blue or hazel eyes and may also have freckles. They tend to tan slowly and with difficulty, as they burn easily. Someone with this type of skin who is unused to direct sunlight will burn after 30 minutes of midsummer sunshine in the UK.

3 The majority of white people have fair skin and are blond or brunette. Their skin will tan given time, but will also burn if the process is rushed. Eye colour is a good indicator of sensitivity. Pale-skinned dark-eyed people tend to tan more readily than those with blue, grey or green eyes — who are at greater risk of burning. Someone with this type of skin who is unused to direct sunlight will burn after 30 minutes of midsummer sunshine.

4 People from China, Japan or the Mediterranean tan much more easily. But they can also burn. Their skin colour ranges from olive to brown and they usually have dark hair and eyes. Their skin may become pale if they stay out of the sun for long periods. Someone with this type of skin who is unused to sunlight will burn after 50 minutes of direct midsummer sunshine in the UK.

5 People from India, South America and Arabia tan well and rarely burn. They have dark skin and hair and brown or black eyes. However, someone with this type of skin who is unused to sunlight will burn after about 70 minutes of direct midsummer sunshine in the UK.

6 Most people with brown to black Afro-Caribbean skin and hair can spend long periods in the sun with little risk of burning. Sunlight does not readily penetrate or damage dark skin, because the high melanin content filters out most of its ultraviolet component.

Of course, your body's response to sunlight is influenced by many more factors than skin type and the time of year when you exposed yourself to the sun's rays. Your age, state of health, diet and medication can have a profound effect on the outcome of sunbathing. So too do a number of other factors such as the time of day when you sunbathe, the amount of skin you expose, how far you are from the equator, how high you are above sea level, how much pollution there is in the atmosphere, how much cloud cover is present, what fabrics you are wearing, air movement over your body, the amount of solar radiation that is reflected onto you from nearby surfaces and so on. This is why guidelines on sunbathing are so difficult to formulate and the task is not made any easier by some of the rather contradictory recommendations put forward by experts in different fields of public health. So before we examine the sun's impact on other aspects of our physical and mental wellbeing, it might be instructive to review some of the available advice on sunbathing and vitamin D given to us by the experts.

The overriding concern of skin specialists involved in the ongoing debate on sunlight and health is to reduce the number of deaths from skin cancer. One of the more influential bodies in this field is the UK Skin Cancer Prevention Working Party whose *Consensus Statement*, published in 1997, stresses the risks to the skin of exposure to the sun. The authors of this document advise both children and adults to protect themselves from the sun; particularly during periods of sunny weather during the spring and early summer. Their *Consensus Statement* makes it quite clear that a tan is not safe, that tanned skin is not a sign of health and offers no more than minimal protection against further exposure. They put forward a four point plan to moderate skin damage caused by sunlight:

- avoid the sun between the hours of 11 a.m. and 3 p.m.
- seek natural shade
- use clothing as a sunscreen, such as T-shirts, long sleeved shirts and hats
- use broad spectrum sunscreens to protect against UVA and UVB radiation

Fairly straightforward you might think. Well, perhaps not if you want to maintain adequate vitamin D levels in your body, because the effects of this sort of behaviour on vitamin D status have not been researched.

In 1998 the UK Department of Health published a report entitled *Nutrition and Bone Health,* which deals with vitamin D and calcium intake amongst the British public. The authors of this report called for the beneficial and adverse effects of sunlight exposure to be reviewed, and for guidelines which strike a balance between reducing the risk of skin cancer and maintaining adequate levels of vitamin D amongst the British population. They asserted in this report that the majority of the adult population in Britain can obtain all of the vitamin D they need if the skin of the face and arms is exposed for about half an hour each day between April and October.

Now, clearly, the Skin Cancer Prevention Working Party's recommendations rather limit opportunities to synthesise vitamin D in this way. On the other hand, the face and arms are the parts of the body which are most susceptible to skin cancer and photoageing. So how does one square the circle? One way is to examine how sunlight was used to cure diseases years ago and compare what was known then with what we know today about the various factors that influence sunbathing. But, for the moment, we will continue to examine the beneficial effects of sunlight on the human body.

SUNLIGHT AND THE BLOOD

Sunlight penetrates far enough into our skin to irradiate the blood passing through the capillaries that lie near the surface. In medical literature published in Eastern Europe there are reports that the electrocardiogram readings and blood profiles of patients with atherosclerosis (hardening of the arteries) improves when they are exposed to ultraviolet radiation. Also, studies have shown that exposure to sunlight, or ultraviolet radiation from an artificial source, increases the number of white blood cells in human blood. The white cells which increase the most are called lymphocytes and these play a major role in defending the body against infections. Sunlight also increases both the oxygen content of human blood and its capacity to deliver oxygen to the tissues, in much the same way that regular exercise does. Significantly, research shows that exercise combined with exposure to the sun has a greater effect on stamina, fitness and muscular development than exercise alone. The ancient Greeks used to exercise in the nude — presumably for this reason — and our word gymnasium comes from the Greek word *gymnasion* which means 'a place for naked exercise or training'. Regular exercise also lowers blood sugar levels — and so does sunlight. This is not particularly noticeable in normal individuals, but is quite marked in diabetics who normally have to take insulin to keep their blood sugar down. The amount of insulin they need to maintain normal blood sugar levels can change significantly if they exercise or are in strong sunlight for any length of time.

Exposure to sunlight also speeds up the elimination of toxic chemicals from the body. This is most obvious in premature babies who are particularly susceptible to jaundice. The blood of jaundiced babies becomes contaminated with a compound called bilirubin. Normally bilirubin is removed by the liver and excreted from the body. But when the liver is not fully functional, as is often the case with new-born or prematurely born infants, bilirubin in the blood can rise to dangerous levels. Years ago infant jaundice could only be treated by blood transfusions, and sometimes blood had to be exchanged three or four times, which could be hazardous.

One sign that there is an excess of bilirubin in the blood is that the skin takes on a characteristic yellowness. In 1956 a nurse in charge of a premature baby unit at the Rochford Hospital, Essex, in England made a remarkable discovery. On warm summer days the nurse, Sister Ward, would wheel babies out of her premature infant unit and into a south-facing courtyard. She was of the 'old school', believing that the combination of fresh air and warm sunshine would do them more good than the stuffy overheated atmosphere of an incubator. She noticed that when she put jaundiced babies out in the sun their skin returned to its normal colour. Researchers who investigated Sister Ward's improvised sunlight therapy found that the blue portion of the visible spectrum was particularly effective in breaking down bilirubin in babies' blood, and in the years that followed it became standard procedure to give 'blue light treatment' from an artificial source, rather than sunlight. Although it is much more convenient for hospital staff to put a baby under a lamp than to take it outside into the sunlight, the latter is more natural. Mothers are now being discouraged from putting babies out in the sun and this may not be in the best interests of the child, as research suggests that exposure to sunlight in infancy protects against disease in later life, a subject examined in Chapter 3.

SUNLIGHT AND GROWTH

Each of us responds differently to sunlight — even in the womb — as a recent study in the journal *Nature* illustrates. Seasonal variations in light levels are known to regulate reproduction and growth in mammals. One of the more striking discoveries about the effects of sunlight on human development is that children born in the spring tend to be taller when they become adults than children born in the autumn. Researchers at the University of Vienna's Institute of Human Biology have shown that the month of birth and, in particular, variation of sunlight levels in the latter stages of pregnancy influence growth to adulthood.

Over a ten-year period more than half a million conscripts to the Austrian Federal Army were examined and an analysis of their body heights revealed a clear link between month of birth and height at 18 years of age. Average body heights were found to vary over a 365 day period, and this pronounced annual rhythm had a synchronous relationship with light levels from the sun. Height peaked at the beginning of April and fell to its lowest point at the beginning of October, while sunlight reached its maximum in July and minimum in January. In humans, growth is fastest during the three months before and after birth. One explanation for the close association between growth and the sun found in this study is that the duration of sunlight during this critical period may regulate the amount of growth hormone in the blood stream of the mother, and then the infant.

In northern Europe there is a long tradition of June weddings; and the annual celebration of the May King and Queen reinforces this custom. A child conceived in June or July would be born in the spring, when sunlight duration is gradually increasing. A child born in the autumn, on the other hand, would have to spend far more time indoors during its first six months. In ancient times this would have reduced its chances of survival as, being inside in the winter, it would be more likely to pick up respiratory infections and have low levels of vitamin D during this formative period. So these old fertility rites may have been introduced to try and encourage spring births and so reduce infant mortality. There is, in fact, a famous reference to the influence of the sun on conception and pregnancy which comes from ancient Egypt. It is part of a *Hymn to the Sun* written by the Pharaoh Akhenaten of the Eighteenth Dynasty (1353–1337 BC) and is quoted in the book *Man and the Sun* by Jacquetta Hawkes, as follows:

> *Boats sail upstream and boats sail downstream,*
> *At your coming every highway is opened.*
> *Before your face the fish leap up from the river,*
> *Your rays reach the green ocean.*
> *You it is who place the male seed in woman,*
> *Who create the semen in man;*
> *You quicken the son in his mother's belly,*
> *Soothing him so that he shall not cry.*
> *Even in the womb you are his nurse.*
> *You give breath to all your creation,*
> *Opening the mouth of the newborn*
> *And giving him nourishment.*

In his hymn, Akhenaten explains how the universe has been made by a sun-god and how all life comes from him. Indeed, Akhenaten has been described as the first sunlight therapist, because he showed an unusual reverence for the life and health-giving power of the sun and was depicted with his beautiful queen, Nefertiti, holding up their young daughters to its rays. During Akhenaten's reign the sun was shown radiating beams, some of which bring the 'ankh', the hieroglyphic signifying 'life', to the royal couple.

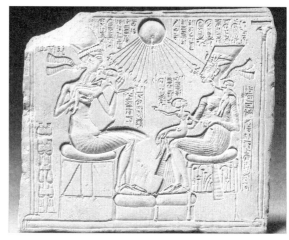

Figure 1: Limestone relief of the Pharaoh Akhenaten and Queen Nefertiti holding up their daughters to the life-giving rays of the sun

Akhenaten is better known as one of history's great heretics because, when he came to power, he broke with the past by announcing that there was only one god, the sun-god Aten. His revolutionary solar cult was a significant forerunner of later monotheistic religion. It was also entirely different from the worship of Ra, Horus, Isis, Osiris and the other Egyptian gods, in that no human or animal form was ever attached to it. However, shortly after Akhenaten's death the old gods were restored. Tutenkamun became Pharaoh and Egypt reverted to the traditional forms of sun-worship which had been practised for the previous sixteen centuries. Akhenaten's reign, his name and his very existence were erased from the annals of Egyptian history. Akhenaten's revolutionary sun-worship came to a rather unhappy end, but at least we still have his hymn in praise of the sun.

THE PSYCHOLOGY OF THE SUN

Western literature is littered with references to the sun and its capacity to lift the spirits. Writers, especially poets, have commented on this over and over again. Yet it is only since the 1980s that the link between light deprivation and depressive illness has been scientifically proven. Of course, the idea that sadness and despair can be triggered by low light levels during the winter months is not new to the medical profession. In 4th century BC, Hippocrates, the 'Father of Medicine', wrote that medical students should investigate the seasons and what occurs in them, because of their influence on physical and mental health. Practitioners of oriental medicine have always examined the effects of the different seasons on their patients. But the condition which is now called seasonal affective disorder (SAD), a form of depression that comes on during the winter months, has until recently gone largely unrecognized and undiagnosed in the West.

One reason for the occurrence of SAD is that the buildings in which we spend our time often force us to live independently of the seasons. If this were not bad enough, we also spend our time indoors at low light levels. Few modern offices, factories and shopping centres admit sunlight and daylight to any great extent, and, as we shall see in the next chapter, artificial light is a poor substitute for the sun's rays. The seasonless, perpetual twilight of the late 20th century is not what we were designed for, which may explain why seasonal affective disorder is so common. It is said to affect 1-3 per cent of the UK population, with a further 20 per cent experiencing a milder form of the condition.

Outdoor light levels are the ones under which we evolved. The intensity of illumination outdoors is several orders of magnitude greater than that provided by artificial lighting. In modern buildings electric lights provide somewhere between 150 and 600 lux, while outside, at noon, sunshine can deliver 100,000 lux. In a sunlit room there can be as many as 60,000 lux falling on a plain surface. Even outside on an overcast, rainy winter day, at northerly latitudes, light intensities of 1000 lux are common for six hours or more.

Patients with SAD have, until recently, received artificial light treatment at about 2,500 lux, but it is becoming more common to treat SAD with shorter exposures at 10,000 lux. But a study published in the *Journal of Affective Disorders*, in 1996, has shown that during the winter months the symptoms of SAD can be alleviated simply by taking an hourly walk each morning. This discovery should come as no surprise to anyone who has read Hippocrates or the works of other medical authorities from classical times: exercise outdoors has been advocated as a remedy for melancholy down the ages. What is also clear from reading medical literature from the past is that getting sunlight into buildings has often been promoted as a way of preventing disease, including depression. Yet it is only very recently that scientific research has shown this to be the case. In another article published in the *Journal of Affective Disorders* in 1996, it was reported that clinically depressed patients in sunny hospital rooms fare better than those in dull rooms. Patients with severe non-seasonal depression at a psychiatric hospital who were lucky enough to be put in sunlit rooms and, as a consequence, got involuntary light treatment from the sun via their windows were discharged more quickly than patients in rooms which received no direct sunlight. The findings of this study bear out what has long been suspected about the importance of getting sunlight into buildings, and the implications will be discussed in due course, but for the moment, let us further explore seasonal affective disorder: what it is, and who gets it.

The sun's daily cycle of light and dark regulates many of the body's most important hormonal and biochemical processes. It is our external timekeeper. It keeps our internal biological clock running smoothly. Without the time-cues, or 'zeitgebers', given by light and dark and, to a lesser extent, by the normal daily routines of breakfast, work, lunchtime, bedtime and so on, the underlying rhythm of the human body reverts to a cycle which is closer to twenty-five hours than twenty-four. So, left to its own devices our internal clock 'free runs' and adds about forty minutes each day. After twenty days of free running, with forty minutes added each day, the normal pattern of waking and sleeping is reversed. Sleep takes place during the day, and the waking hours are at night. This is a pattern which is sometimes seen in people whose circadian rhythms are disturbed because of blindness or Alzheimer's disease.

The symptoms that distinguish SAD from non-seasonal clinical depression include overeating, a craving for carbohydrates, and weight gain during the autumn and winter months. During the spring, a SAD sufferer may also find that their depression is replaced by mild hypomania and marked changes in energy levels, sleep patterns and eating habits. Seasonal affective disorder is usually diagnosed when depression occurs at the same time each year on three or more occasions. So, if you have no recollection of this, you are not a SAD sufferer in the strict sense.

If you find out that you are suffering from SAD, what can you do about it? The first step is to arrange an appointment with a consultant who can make a full diagnosis and give guidance on treatment, which will depend on the severity of the condition. It may consist of drugs, light, or a combination of the two. The symptoms of SAD can be relieved by light therapy, but the reasons for this are not clearly understood. It seems that light may act on the neurohormones in the brain that govern mood and behaviour. How and why this happens is still something of a mystery: there is no general consensus as to how light therapy works. Relief from the symptoms can follow relatively short exposures to light at 10,000 lux, and for some sufferers this form of treatment is most effective immediately after waking. But the condition can also be alleviated with a device known as a dawn simulator: an alarm clock that works with light rather than sound. Dawn simulators produce a very gradual increase in light levels — to a maximum output of between 200 and 500 lux — in the period immediately before waking. Dawn simulation is effective for SAD sufferers even though their eyes are closed. Indeed, the light intensities used in dawn simulators have been shown to be ineffective on SAD patients when they are fully awake. It may be that dawn simulation is a powerful 'zeitgeber' that triggers some sort of 'wake-up' response in the body which restores the normal hormonal cycle. At some time in our evolutionary past we must have developed a particularly sensitive mechanism for detecting sunrise and this can be used to good effect in the treatment of SAD. Clearly this is very different from bright light therapy, which works directly through the eyes, and so there may be more than one mechanism at work when light therapy is used to treat seasonal depression.

When light enters the eye and stimulates the retina, two things happen. First, nerve impulses travel along the optic nerve to the part of the brain that interprets what we see. At the same time, some nerve impulses pass from the optic nerve to a gland in the brain, the hypothalamus. This gland secretes seratonin, a hormone that plays a key role in controlling moods and regulating sleep patterns, body temperature, digestion and sex drive. Recent research suggests that SAD sufferers have some sort of abnormality in the hypothalamus, which bright light can reverse. Seratonin levels in the hypothalamus fall during the winter months, and low seratonin levels have been linked to anxiety and depression. Indeed, some of the recently developed antidepressants, such as Prozac, alleviate symptoms by increasing seratonin levels in the brain. So bright light treatment may be effective in the treatment of SAD because it rectifies a fundamental seratonin deficiency.

One of the functions of seratonin is to suppress the secretion of another neurohormone, melatonin, which is produced by the pineal gland. When light levels fall, seratonin production declines and the pineal begins to secrete melatonin into the bloodstream. Melatonin induces sleep by depressing activity in the brain and slowing down other physiological processes. It acts as the 'master hormone' stimulating the release of hormones from other glands, including the pituitary, adrenals, ovaries and testes. These, in turn, regulate a number of bodily processes, from digestion and menstruation to the onset of puberty.

A few years ago melatonin was being hailed as a wonder drug because it was thought that many age-related health problems were caused by declining levels of melatonin in the body, and that oral supplements of melatonin could be used to offset this decline and slow down the ageing process. Boosting levels of the hormone in this way was supposed to have a number of beneficial effects including: improving sleep; stimulating the immune system; lowering blood pressure; and preventing cancer. Melatonin is available over the counter in some countries, although it has been withdrawn from sale in the UK. The jury appears still to be out as far as the medicinal and anti-ageing properties of melatonin are concerned, although it is used to alter disrupted sleep patterns. But, leaving aside melatonin, seratonin, and the effects of these hormones on the body, let us look a little more closely at sunlight and depression.

Depression is a very common illness, affecting as much as 10 per cent of the UK population at any one time. It is the most frequently diagnosed symptom, and the cause of more hospital admissions than any other psychiatric disorder. Vast sums have been, and continue to be, spent on this distressing and sometimes life-threatening condition. The World Health Organization estimate that the annual cost of depression in the United States is $44 billion, equal to the total cost of all cardiovascular diseases. As we have already seen, light therapy seems to have a beneficial effect on non-seasonal depression, and if you spend your time in a sunlit room your recovery can be more rapid than if you stay in a dark room. One could be forgiven for thinking that this was common knowledge, and that psychiatric wards for the treatment of depressed patients would be designed to let the sun in. After all, this relatively simple measure would save a fortune in drugs, and in the care and supervision of patients. But it does not appear to have been a priority for designers — to everyone's cost. In fact, there have been few incentives for designers and planners to create sunlit spaces for health; even though many people from antiquity onwards recognized that getting sunlight into buildings might have a favourable impact on the psychological wellbeing of occupants. The Roman philosopher and writer Aulus Cornelius Celsus (25 BC–AD 50) advised sufferers of melancholy to live in rooms 'full of light'. Opportunities for their modern day counterparts to do so have been rather limited by the way buildings have been designed.

It should be said that, as with other forms of illness, depression can be made worse by exposing sufferers to bright light, or to the sun. As Dorothy Rowe explains in her book on depression *Breaking the Bonds*, this is not due to any physiological effect but, rather, to the significance the sun holds for the sufferer:

> *… not everybody feels more cheerful in sunshine. People who are depressed can find sunshine very difficult, and there is always a rise in the suicide rate in spring. The reason for this is*

*not the effect of sunlight on our bodies but the meaning that
we give to such light. If you value and accept yourself and look
forward optimistically, then spring is always full of promise, but
if you don't value yourself and you expect that only bad things
will happen to you because you are bad, then spring is not full
of promise but only threats.*

WINTER BLUES AND LIGHT HUNGER

A substantial proportion of the UK population — possibly as much as 20 per cent
— may suffer from a mild form of depression in the winter months: the so-called
'winter blues'. Again, this may well be because they spend very little time
outdoors, or are confined in buildings that admit very little sunlight during the
winter. In addition to this form of mild depression there is another disorder that
may be caused by modern lifestyles, which is referred to as 'light hunger'. One
symptom that is sometimes commented on when SAD is being discussed is that
sufferers express a craving for light, or need to turn lights on at every opportunity.
As the great light therapist and Nobel Laureate Dr Niels Finsen remarked in an
interview in 1903, the year before he died:

> *All that I have accomplished in my experiments with light and
> all that I have learned about its therapeutic value has come
> because I needed the light so much myself. I longed for it so.*

A lot of other people do too, judging by the way they behave when they are
on holiday at a sunny resort. By baking themselves in the midday sun, they may
well be trying to make up for lost time, or lost sunlight. This behaviour could be
a manifestation of 'light hunger', the body crying out for light as Niels Finsen
described, no matter how harmful that light may be to the skin. As with seasonal
affective disorder, the sunburn that is the inevitable consequence of 'bingeing' on
sunlight may have its origins in the buildings we inhabit, and the inordinate
amount of time we spend in them. Even if you don't normally sunbathe, there is
a very good case for spending an hour each day out of doors year-round to
maintain your psychological wellbeing and, if your eyesight is defective,
preferably without your glasses on or contact lenses in place.

Glass filters out wavelengths below 350 nm, which means that no UVB
radiation, and only a limited amount of UVA, passes through. This explains why
you cannot get a tan behind window glass. As the lenses in spectacles also filter

out these wavelengths, they prevent the full spectrum of natural light reaching the retina at the back of the eye. The human eye evolved to accommodate the full spectrum of the sun's rays and it seems reasonable to suggest, as some researchers do, that the full spectrum of sunlight is what it should be exposed to. But, before we go much further, a cautionary note. Never look into the sun, or at an eclipse of the sun, as this will cause permanent damage to the eye. In the days before navigational aids of any sophistication, blindness was an occupational hazard for sailors and explorers. These mariners of old found their latitude with 'sighting sticks' which were used to measure the height of the sun above the horizon. They had to stare directly at the sun to record its position and get their bearings, a practice which cost them some or all of their eyesight.

There is a striking irony surrounding the developments related to SAD and light therapy. On the one hand people spend so much time indoors that they are investing in light-boxes and dawn simulators to compensate for lack of sunlight, and on the other they are being discouraged from going out into the sun at all. Of course, there is no connection between SAD and sunbathing. Or is there? Well, one of the symptoms of vitamin D deficiency is depression, and it has been suggested that the seasonal nature and symptoms of SAD may be due changes in levels of vitamin D_3 leading to changes in seratonin levels. Indeed the author of a paper in the journal *Medical Hypothesis*, published in 1998, went so far as to suggest that the amount of serotonin produced in winter may be dependent on the amount of light exposure the previous summer. So here is evidence, albeit limited, that sunbathing during the summer months may have psychological as well as physiological effects in the winter. If this is the case, then the light therapy used on SAD sufferers may simply be compensating for low levels of serotonin brought on by lack of sunlight in the summer. It would certainly be interesting to conduct an experiment to see whether summer sunbathing prevents winter depression. But, clearly, this would run counter to the spirit of current health campaigns advocating avoidance of the sun.

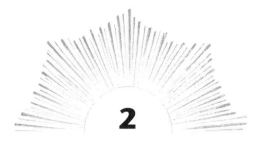

2

THE DECLINE OF THE SUN

From the earliest agricultural civilizations onwards, the passage of time has been calculated according to natural cycles. Knowledge of the seasons allowed our ancestors to plan the sowing and reaping of crops. It helped them to manage their livestock and to anticipate the migration of wild game. By studying the phases of the moon they could work out when floodwaters would return to irrigate the land; and when they could hold religious celebrations and social occasions at night and still be able to see each other. Religious leaders and kings were sometimes chosen because they were supposed to be able to exert a favourable influence on the sun and produce good harvests and good weather for gathering in crops. When they failed, they risked being sacrificed — or someone else did.

Natural cycles were also studied because they were felt to have a profound influence on health, but today the inhabitants of developed countries don't need to know anything about the cycles of the sun and moon. Our increasingly urban world means that we can, if we so wish, shield ourselves from the changing seasons and contact with the sun. However, the experiences of physicians from other cultures and other periods in history suggests that such isolation may be detrimental to our health and wellbeing, as we shall see.

In the ancient world, sun-gods and goddesses were often worshipped as deities of medicine. They performed miracles of healing, and brought enlightenment and truth. But they could also be vengeful and destructive. It seems our ancestors were only too well aware that there was a dark as well as a light side to the sun, and that both aspects were worthy of their respect. The sun was central to their lives and, as they had to attune themselves to its natural cycles in order to survive, they were probably much better equipped to know when sunlight was harmful and when it was beneficial than we are. Nevertheless, our physiological and psychological requirements are much the same as theirs. We thrive on, and are strengthened by, the stimulus of change, and are weakened by monotony — and one of the greatest agents of change in our lives is the sun.

Yet, at the present time we hear rather more about the hazards of sunlight — the dark side — than the benefits. Sunbathing is now portrayed as a social evil comparable to cigarette smoking or alcohol abuse. There is, we are told, no such thing as a healthy tan: a healthy tan is an oxymoron. Given current concerns about skin cancer, especially its most dangerous form malignant melanoma, and the 'hole' in the ozone layer, this is an understandable development. So there are now few obvious incentives to get outdoors and benefit from the positive aspects of the sun and, thanks to modern lifestyles, it is not as easy to attune ourselves to natural cycles as it once was. We can now work, rest, play, shop and travel in an artificial environment, and have very little direct contact with the outside world. One consequence of all this is that, for many of us, sunlight plays only a small part in our daily lives.

It can be quite instructive to sit down with a pen and a piece of paper and work out just how much time you spend indoors each week. Some estimates put the average figure at about 90 per cent, and if you work at home, or are sick or elderly or of pre-school age the figure can be higher. This is in marked contrast to our ancestors, most of whom would have been working on the land from dawn until dusk for much of the year. From what we have already seen in the previous chapter, if you don't go out in the summer sunshine the levels of vitamin D in your body could be rather lower than required, and you may also be at risk of seasonal depression. But there other disadvantages to spending many hours each day indoors, especially in buildings which do not admit much sunlight or daylight, and are illuminated artificially.

ARTIFICIAL INDOOR LIGHT

The way that buildings are designed and, especially, the way they are lit can have a profound influence the physical and psychological wellbeing of their occupants. Ideally, the artificial lighting to which you expose yourself day in and day out, should be as close as possible to the lighting environment under which your ancestors evolved, the solar spectrum. Unfortunately, artificial lighting is not designed in this way. It has been developed under the assumption that the only significant purpose of light for humans is to enable us to see. The lighting industry has not addressed our biological needs, but simply satisfies our most basic visual requirements. Indeed, one of the deciding factors in the choice of lighting for offices, factories, shops and public spaces is energy efficiency rather than health.

The spectral distribution of the colours produced by artificial lighting differs markedly from that of sunlight. Incandescent lamps — ordinary screw-in light bulbs — emit a large proportion of their output as yellow and red light. Most of the electricity they use is converted into infra-red radiation rather than visible light, which is why they give off so much heat and use a lot of electricity. In contrast, fluorescent lights generate visible light by a non-thermal process and so the tubes remain much cooler and less electricity is needed to run them. Their spectral distribution depends on the type of fluorescent coating they are given. The most widely used are the so-called 'cool-white' fluorescent tubes which generate most of their output as yellow and green light and are deficient at the red and blue-violet ends of the visible spectrum; this is where the output of the sun is strongest. They produce an alternating light output or near-subliminal 'flicker' which has been shown to be a source of stress for building users — and an extremely low output of ultraviolet radiation. Some manufacturers will supply so-called 'full-spectrum' fluorescent tubes which are much closer to the natural spectrum and produce a small amount of ultraviolet radiation. Now available too are incandescent bulbs which achieve a much closer match, but they do not have an ultraviolet component in their output. For the most part we now live and work in a lighting environment that is unnatural and does not produce in us the same photochemical responses that natural daylight does.

Unlike artificial lighting with its static output, the brightness and colour of daylight is continually changing in a building from sunrise to sunset, because of the sun's apparent movement, cloud formation and shadows. The intensity of light is also generally much greater. So by getting daylight into living spaces you are creating a healthier environment, because it is more natural. Daylight normally enters from the side of a building, whereas the fluorescent lighting used in schools, offices and factories generally radiates from above. So, if there is little or no daylight, or sunlight penetration, fluorescent lighting can produce a shadowless, monotonous environment. If fluorescent lights are installed in a room with a white ceiling and white walls, there will be a lot of reflection and re-reflection. Everything is brightly lit but there is no depth, which is decidedly unnatural. Moreover, in the absence of daylight, there will be no time cues or zeitgebers to help synchronize your body clock. In addition, light levels may well be at or near those of natural twilight and will not suppress melatonin secretion.

Evidence is emerging which suggests that the long-term effects of artificial 'light pollution' may be harmful: as the following examples illustrate. One of the hormones secreted by the pituitary gland stimulates the adrenal gland. The pituitary gland will overproduce this adrenal-stimulating hormone if lighting conditions differ markedly from the natural spectrum. In one study a comparison of the effects of exposure to natural light and artificial light on the amount of adrenocorticotrophic hormone (ACTH) secreted into the bloodstream gave a clear indication of this. A fortnight spent in 'cool-white' fluorescent light at about 3,500 lux increased the ACTH levels in test subjects to abnormally high levels, resulting in stress. Their ACTH levels returned to normal after two weeks of exposure to daylight. When the experiment was carried out with full-spectrum lighting instead of the 'cool white' lights, there was a significantly lower level of the 'stress hormone' ACTH in the blood. So, bright artificial light which is different in its spectral composition from sunlight puts stress on the body in as short a period as two weeks. On this basis it is clear that while we can relax on holiday in sunshine at 50,000 lux, artificial light at these levels would be very disturbing indeed. Dr Fritz Hollwich, who carried out this research, and discussed the results in his book of 1979, *The Influence of Ocular Light Perception on Metabolism on Man and in Animal,* concluded that:

> Natural light, involving the whole body, is a vital element like
> water and air. As such, it should accompany the human
> individual for as many hours of the day as the course of the
> seasons permits.

Prolonged exposure to artificial light at normal levels may compromise the immune system in, as yet, unknown ways. A potential risk factor for malignant melanoma which is not perhaps as well known as it might be is prolonged exposure to ordinary fluorescent lighting. Epidemiological, clinical and animal studies suggest that this common form of illumination, which was introduced into the workplace in the 1950s, is associated with melanoma. The link may not be that strong, but it should not be lightly dismissed. Another potential problem faced by indoor workers is that the synthesis of vitamin D in the skin does not occur under electric lights, or behind window glass. Several studies have shown that vitamin D levels in people who live and work exclusively in a conventional artificially lit environment fall markedly with time. For anyone who spends long periods indoors and cannot get sunlight exposure on a regular basis, full-spectrum lights might be a useful addition to their lighting regime.

COMFORT AND HEALTH

The human body has temperature control mechanisms which exist to compensate for changes in the environment. They keep the internal temperature of the body at the right level and are designed to accommodate the continual, gradual changes in temperature and humidity normally experienced outdoors. Our ability to respond to variations in temperature and humidity is compromised if we constantly live and work in conditions that do not change. Central heating and air-conditioning systems create indoor environments that stay within close limits to keep us comfortable. But sacrificing the stimulus of change for comfort in this way may not be beneficial to our health. Also, moving to and from interiors that are maintained at levels of temperature and humidity markedly different from those outdoors may be prejudicial to our wellbeing. In crude terms this sort of sudden transition from a cold environment to a hot one, or vice versa, is rather like changing one season for another. It is worth noting that practitioners of some traditional forms of medicine regard the days in which seasonal changes occur (from winter to spring, spring to summer, etc.) as being the times of year when the human body is at its most vulnerable to sickness and infection. They consider sudden changes of season as particularly unwelcome.

The human body needs the challenge of gradually changing conditions, and regular exercise, if it is to be strong and healthy. The more active you are, the more food you can consume without getting fat. If you are engaged in hard manual work in cool conditions you can eat plenty of food and not put on weight. It requires far fewer calories to sustain a modern sedentary lifestyle. A recent dietary and nutritional survey of British adults showed that on average they eat about 10 per cent less than the amount that is still recognized as the norm: 2,000 calories a day for women and 2,500 for men. The British are burning fewer calories and are getting fatter, and this is probably because they are getting less and less active and more and more comfortable. Only 20 per cent of men and 10 per cent of women are now employed in active occupations. In the UK we now watch an average of 28 hours of TV each week, which is twice the amount we were watching in the 1960s.

Obesity increased amongst the UK population from 8 per cent in 1980, to 15 per cent in 1995. In the United States it has reached the level of an epidemic. Some 20 per cent of American men and 24 per cent of American women were classified as obese in 1994, and the incidence is increasing. Obesity is also a major health problem amongst the more affluent populations in developing countries who adopt the western way of life. Anyone who is 20 per cent, or more, over the

41

maximum desirable weight for their height is obese, rather than simply overweight. As such, they are susceptible to a number of chronic conditions such as diabetes, gall-stones, arterial disease, high blood pressure, and respiratory disease. The increase in obesity worldwide is a major public health issue, not least because of the enormous burden of disability and death which will be associated with it in the longer term.

The body's mechanisms for regulating body weight function much more effectively on a low fat, high carbohydrate diet, and the intake of fat in British and American diets has increased steadily since the 1940s. But there is a much closer relationship between low levels of physical activity and obesity than there is between obesity and diet. So, buildings that encourage sedentary lifestyles pose a threat to the health of their occupants, and this seems to have been appreciated rather more widely at the beginning of the 20th century than is the case at present. The reasons for this are examined later in chapter 6, which is concerned with the indoor environment, health, and the sun.

OZONE DEPLETION AND SUNBATHING

An issue of great concern to scientists, politicians and sunbathers is the possibility that ultraviolet radiation is becoming more harmful. The ultraviolet component of sunlight is divided into three categories depending on wavelength: near-UV or UVA radiation; mid-UV or UVB radiation; and far-UV or UVC radiation. All of the UVC radiation and much of this UVB radiation is absorbed by ozone in the earth's upper atmosphere. Following the discovery by the British Antarctic Survey in 1985 that there was a 'hole' in the ozone layer over the Antarctic, there has been speculation that an increase in UVB radiation, due to ozone depletion by CFCs (chlorofluorocarbons) and other chemicals, would cause health problems. But the much feared, and publicized, consequences that have been predicted for the decline in ozone have not so far been observed. There have been no increases in skin cancers, eye diseases, immune system disorders or environmental damage which can be attributed to an increase in ultraviolet radiation.

The largest South American city close to the Antarctic ozone hole is Punta Arenas in Southern Chile. Despite reports to the contrary, there have been no ozone depletion-related health problems at Punta Arenas, and measurements of ultraviolet radiation, reported in the *American Journal of Public Health* in 1995, show that any increases are too small to have any appreciable effect. A paper published in 1998 by the European Science and Environmental Forum challenges the consensus view on ozone depletion, and argues that predictions made by the scientific establishment and the media have been ill-founded. If this is the case, and the hole in the ozone layer is, after all, a temporary thinning of the upper atmosphere in the early spring, then there is no reason to fear that people will develop skin cancer because ultraviolet radiation has become more dangerous.

There is certainly no evidence to support the widely held view that the increase in malignant melanoma in recent years is in some way linked to ozone depletion. The trend predates the issue of ozone loss, which may have been going on for some time before it was noticed. A paper published in the *British Journal of Cancer* entitled 'The Relationship Between Skin Cancers, Solar Radiation and Ozone Depletion' shows that from 1957 to 1984 the incidence of malignant melanoma in Norway increased by 350 per cent for men and 440 per cent for women. During the same period there was no change in ozone levels over Norway nor any significant change in annual exposure to ultraviolet radiation from the sun.

Scare stories, such as the one about sheep in Chile developing cataracts because of increased ultraviolet radiation, are not supported in the scientific literature. The sheep in question were later found to have had an infectious disease, and sunlight was not implicated. What is clear, however, is that there is a great deal of ill-informed comment on the subject of ozone depletion and, for that matter, sunbathing. Should depletion of the ozone layer ever become a cause for real concern, then some people might develop cancer who might not have, had there been no depletion, but until this happens there is much more to be gained from investigating the real causes of skin cancer and encouraging safe sunbathing than in being preoccupied with the state of the earth's upper atmosphere and blaming everything on the sun. Diet and lifestyle play a far more significant part in the genesis of cancer than is currently recognized. The same can also be said about another condition that is supposed to be on the increase because of ozone depletion — that of senile cataract.

SUNLIGHT AND CATARACTS

It is clear from a number of studies that if you live in a sunny part of the world you are more likely to develop cataracts in old age than if you live in a less sunny region. In much the same way that sunbathing is now being actively discouraged, experts are now saying that exposure of the eye to ultraviolet radiation is dangerous and steps should be taken to avoid it. We are advised to wear sunglasses which block the UV component of the sun's rays, just as we are advised to wear sunscreens and sunblocks on our skin to prevent skin cancer.

This is, of course, unnatural. The human eye evolved in sunlight and is well equipped to cope with its full spectrum. Sunglasses are, for the most part, a fashion accessory. Our ancestors managed quite well without them. If at any time they felt the need to protect their eyes from the glare of the sun they put on a hat or stayed in the shade. Aldous Huxley, in his book *The Art of Seeing,* recalled that in his youth it was assumed that anyone seen wearing tinted glasses or goggles did so because they were blind or had a problem with their sight. There was a considerable stigma attached to wearing anything of this sort: it certainly was not considered fashionable or desirable. What has happened during the last forty years or so is that people have stopped wearing hats as a matter of course, and have taken to wearing sunglasses. This may be because they spend less time outdoors than they used to and their eyes have difficulty coping with natural levels of daylight and sunlight. But the burning question is 'does solar radiation actually cause cataracts?'

During the early years of the 20th century it became clear that cataracts were far more common in third-world countries than in the West, and this led to the 'sunlight hypothesis' of caractogenesis. This hypothesis, which ignored differences in diet, culture, poverty, malnutrition and disease — and proposed solar radiation as the sole cause — survives to this day. Yet ultraviolet radiation has never been shown to cause cataracts in humans. A causal relationship has never been established, although many researchers have tried to do so. In fact, there have been a number of studies which provide powerful evidence against the sunlight hypothesis of cataracts; and several other possible causes have been put forward in place of solar radiation. One suggestion is that severe diarrhoea could account for the excess cataracts in the Third World, as this diarrhoea leads to severe demineralization of the body. There are other aspects of poor living conditions, such as malnutrition, smoking and pollution that have been proposed as factors contributory to cataracts. Strong sunlight will cause damage to the eyes in other ways. It only takes about two hours of exposure around midday in snow-covered terrain for photokeratitis, otherwise known as snow-blindness, to develop. This condition can also be induced in the desert after six to eight hours of exposure. The eye cannot adapt to strong ultraviolet radiation in the way that skin does. Repeated exposure can cause inflammation, swelling and ulceration which is why protective lenses should be worn in extreme conditions.

SKIN CANCER

For the past decade or so health experts have been advising us not to sunbathe, because of the increasing incidence of skin cancer. The number of cases of malignant melanoma, the most serious form of the disease, are increasing and, as a result, major health education programmes have been set up to warn people of the dangers of sunbathing. There are over 4000 new cases in the UK each year, while in the United States some 40,000 cases were diagnosed in 1998. It is widely accepted that there is a causal link between the sun's ultraviolet radiation and malignant melanoma, and that the increase in rates of skin cancer is due to the way sunbathing is now practised. Sunlight exposure can, indeed, lead to premature ageing, the formation of keratin plaques, and other unsightly skin conditions. But what one has to bear in mind is that there are health risks associated with not getting enough sunlight, and these risks may well be more significant than that posed by malignant melanoma.

There seems little doubt that ultraviolet radiation from the sun can cause two types of skin cancer in fair-skinned people: basal cell carcinoma and squamous cell carcinoma. Both respond to treatment in almost all cases and few sufferers die from them. Squamous cell carcinoma is thought to be the result of cumulative exposure to sunlight, rather than sunburn, and generally develops in old age. Until recently, basal cell carcinoma was also thought to be related to total chronic sun exposure, but there is now substantial evidence that it is actually the intermittent exposure of skin unaccustomed to the sun's rays that is the major causal factor for this form of skin cancer. Malignant melanoma — the much rarer and more lethal skin cancer — affects a younger age-group than either basal or squamous cell cancers, and may be triggered by several episodes of severe sunburn. But its causes are still poorly understood and the exact nature of its relationship with sunlight exposure has yet to be determined.

Basal cell carcinomas, which are also known as 'rodent ulcers', develop on parts of the body which get most exposure to the sun, particularly the face and hands. Unlike other forms of cancer, basal cell carcinomas do not spread to other parts of the body, but if left untreated these small ulcers work their way deeply into underlying tissues causing serious damage and disfigurement. Small carcinomas of this type can be cleared up either by freezing the damaged tissue — cryotherapy — or by applying a cream which contains appropriate drugs. Surgery or radiotherapy may be required for larger lesions.

Squamous cell carcinoma is the second most common form of non-melanoma skin cancer and also tends to develop on the face and hands. It is more dangerous than basal cell carcinoma because it can spread to other parts of the body if left untreated. This form of cancer is linked to damage caused by ultraviolet radiation and exposure to certain industrial chemicals. It appears as red scaly areas which bleed easily and may sometimes ulcerate, and is treated with surgery or radiotherapy.

Basal and squamous cancers increased from 19,000 cases in 1974 to 36,000 in 1989 in the UK and, worldwide, there is now an epidemic of basal cell carcinoma. However, these non-melanoma skin cancers mainly affect older people and respond to treatment in about 95 per cent of cases. So, although they can be very distressing, and may cause disfigurement, they are not generally life-threatening. Malignant melanoma is a very different matter. Melanomas grow and spread through the body very quickly and, unless they are caught early, can be very difficult to treat. They can develop at all ages, but they tend to affect younger people and are more common in women than men. Melanoma appears to run in families. Fair-skinned people with red or blond hair, blue or grey eye colour, with a tendency to freckling, and who burn easily, are most at risk of developing the disease. A third of all melanomas start in a pre-existing mole — the rest start in seemingly normal skin — and the greater the number of moles the higher the risk.

It is people such as administrators and managers, professional people, clerical workers and sales workers who are at risk of developing the disease and not people who work outdoors. Research suggests that this may be because office workers spend long periods indoors and periodically subject themselves to short intense bursts of sunlight for which their bodies are ill-prepared. Melanoma is also associated with several episodes of burning in childhood, but the major risk factor for the disease is skin type: people who have difficulty tanning are at highest risk regardless of whether they have a history of sunburn or not.

Malignant melanoma is primarily a cancer of the skin, but it can develop elsewhere: in the eye and, very rarely, at sites which are not exposed to the sun, such as the rectum, vulva, vagina, mouth, respiratory tract, gastro-intestinal tract and bladder. If, as it seems, these noncutaneous malignant melanomas are not be caused by sunlight exposure then there may be other agents at work. There is, indeed, evidence that the risk of developing malignant melanoma can be influenced by non-solar factors: diet; changes in hormonal status; viruses; drugs; traumas to the skin such as burns or wounds; and some occupations which involve exposure to chemicals.

Another consideration to bear in mind is that while melanoma rates have been increasing amongst populations with pale skin, there has been no corresponding increase amongst dark-skinned populations worldwide. The incidence of malignant melanoma amongst non-Caucasians has been about one-third to one-tenth that among Caucasians and does not appear to be related to sunlight exposure. So, if sunlight does not cause malignant melanoma in dark-skinned people, there is the distinct possibility that non-solar factors are at work amongst others who develop it.

Melanomas can appear on the palms, the soles of the feet, and areas usually covered by clothing such as the legs and back. They seldom occur in outdoor workers and there is evidence that regular moderate sunbathing actually reduces the risk of developing this form of cancer. For example, a study of the incidence of the cancer amongst US Navy personnel between 1974 and 1984, published in the *Archives of Environmental Health,* showed that there was a higher incidence of melanoma amongst sailors who had indoor jobs, such as engine crews, than those who worked outdoors. After testicular cancer, melanoma is the second most common cancer amongst males in the US Navy. Sailors who worked both indoors and outdoors gained most protection from melanoma, having rates some 24 per cent below the US national average for the disease, and this seemed to be due to their exposure to the sun. This supports the findings of other studies which suggest that while severe sunburn may initiate malignant melanoma, regular sunning may actually prevent it.

Skin cancers have increased during the 20th century; a century in which more people live and work indoors than ever before. It is said that in 1900 more than three quarters of the population of the United States worked outdoors but by 1970 less than 10 per cent did. This suggests that, while sunlight exposure may trigger these skin cancers, there may be other underlying factors in our lifestyles which make us susceptible: diet; exposure to ionizing radiation; electromagnetic fields; toxic chemicals in the environment; increased stress; and so on. The widely accepted view that there is a causal link between the sun's ultraviolet radiation and skin cancer, and that the increase in rates of skin cancer over the last forty years is due to the way sunbathing is now practised, may be diverting attention away from the real causative agents. On the other hand, sunbathing has changed during the second half of the 20th century in one important respect: products have become available which allow people with pale skin to prolong their exposure to the sun. Before sunscreens were developed, only tanned skin could withstand strong sunlight for long periods without burning.

In an attempt to halt the rise in skin cancers sunscreens have been, and continue to be, promoted by health experts. Sunscreens do prevent burning. But the public have been encouraged to use them in the absence of any scientific evidence that they prevent malignant melanoma or basal cell carcinoma. Unfortunately there is a growing body of opinion that the widespread use of chemical sunscreens since the 1970s has actually contributed to the rapid increase in melanoma during the last twenty years.

SUNSCREENS AND THE SUN

Although the use of sunscreens is promoted as a public health measure for the prevention of skin cancer, there are very good grounds for avoiding them. Sunscreens enable sunbathers to stay out in the sun for much longer than would be the case if their skin were unprotected, and there is evidence that prolonged exposure of this kind may actually increase the risk of melanoma and non-melanoma skin cancer. Sunscreens are categorized by a sun protection factor, or SPF. In simple terms a product with an SPF of fifteen allows a sunbather to stay in the sun fifteen times longer before burning than if they had no lotion on at all. So if they normally started to burn after twenty minutes in the sun, theoretically a sunscreen with this SPF would allow them to delay the onset of burning for five hours. In practice, the effectiveness of a sunscreen can diminish well before the five hours is up, and you have to put generous amounts on your skin at regular intervals if a high level of protection is to be achieved for any length of time. Also, the SPF only refers to the amount of protection given against UVB radiation, not UVA.

Sunlight which reaches the earth's surface contains two wavelengths which can damage the skin: ultraviolet A, or UVA, and ultraviolet B, or UVB. Both promote tanning and burning. UVB burns skin more rapidly than UVA, but does not penetrate as deeply. Ultraviolet B radiation is implicated in all forms of skin cancer, whereas UVA is thought to be linked to malignant melanoma and to premature ageing. Until a few years ago UVA was thought to be relatively safe, but it is now known that these rays penetrate deeply into the skin, where they can damage collagen and elastin, and cause wrinkles and lines to appear.

The association between UVA and melanoma has been offered as one explanation for the awkward fact that there have been reports of an increased risk of the disease amongst sunscreen users. One explanation put forward for this is that, until recently, sunscreens were far more effective at blocking ultraviolet B than ultraviolet A, because UVA was thought to be safe. So the ratio of UVB to UVA absorbed by the skin of someone using a sunscreen was different from the relative proportions in the natural spectrum of sunlight. A sunbather using one of these predominantly UVB sunscreens would expose themselves to disproportionately higher doses of UVA than would be the case if they had no protection on their skin, and so would be at increased risk of a UVA-induced skin disease such as melanoma. Now whether this hypothesis is correct or not, it serves to illustrate just how these products can give the user a false sense of security.

Two epidemiologists, Drs Frank and Cedric Garland, have been responsible for a number of the studies which suggest that vitamin D from solar exposure may help protect against a number of serious cancers, including malignant melanoma. The Garlands have also put forward the hypothesis that vitamin D may actually help protect the skin against UV damage and that, in the absence of vitamin D in the skin, large amounts of UVA may promote the development of cancers which were originally initiated by sunlight exposure during childhood. As the skin makes vitamin D when exposed to UVB but not UVA radiation, their theory adds weight to the argument against the use of predominantly UVB sunscreens. The Garlands made the following observation about malignant melanoma in the *American Journal of Public Health* in 1992:

> *Worldwide, the countries where chemical sunscreens have been recommended and adopted have experienced the greatest rise in malignant melanoma, with a contemporaneous rise in death rates. In the United States, Canada, Australia, and the Scandinavian countries, melanoma rates have risen steeply in recent decades with the greatest increase occurring after the introduction of sunscreens. Death rates in the United States from melanoma doubled in women and tripled in men between the 1950s and 1990s. The rise in melanoma has been unusually steep in Queensland, Australia, where sunscreens were earliest and most strongly promoted by the medical community. Queensland now has the highest incidence rate of melanoma in the world. In contrast, the rise in melanoma rates was notably delayed elsewhere in Australia, where sunscreens were not promoted until more recently.*

Their hypothesis presupposes that regular sunscreen use prevents the synthesis of vitamin D in the skin and, while there is evidence that it can some experts maintain it does not.

Evidence of the potential dangers of prolonging sunlight exposure through sunscreen use comes from a study published in the *Journal of the National Cancer Institute* in 1998. This showed that children who were frequent users of sunscreens had a significantly higher chance of developing moles and freckles than children who were not. Researchers from the European Institute of Oncology counted the number of 'naevi' (moles or freckles) on 613 children aged between six and seven years, from four European cities. Parents gave each child's history of sunscreen use, sunburn, and any physical protection the children had used on holiday outings. The researchers found that children who were high sunscreen users were spending more time in the sun, and had a higher chance of developing moles on their bodies than non-users. Children who wore clothes in the sun, instead of sunscreens, avoided the sun-induced development of naevi. Since a high naevi count is a strong predictor of malignant melanoma in adulthood, children who use sunscreens, stay out in the sun and develop more moles as a result would be at greater risk of skin cancer in their later years.

Sunscreens usually contain one of two types of protection: either a chemical sun filter to absorb ultraviolet radiation, or a physical sun filter. The latter is an inert material such as titanium oxide, zinc oxide, or talc and works by reflecting ultraviolet rays away from the skin. The active ingredients in chemical sunscreens include p-aminobenzoic acid, methoxycinnamate, benzophenone and other agents which absorb certain wavebands of ultraviolet radiation while letting others through. Sunscreens undergo very rigorous testing before being released on the market, but from time to time ingredients have had to be withdrawn because they either cause adverse reactions or are potentially carcinogenic.

In the late 1970s concerns were expressed about a substance called 5-methoxypsoralen which was included in some chemical sunscreens to promote tanning. These formulations were eventually taken off the market because the 5-methoxypsoralen in them was suspected of having other biological effects besides tanning. It was thought that they might behave similarly to other psoralens, such as 8-methoxypsoralen, which were known to produce chromosomal mutations and to have produced skin cancer, in the presence of light, in mice and humans. A contributor to the *British Medical Journal* in 1979 expressed disquiet about this, as follows:

> *It is with considerable uneasiness that I suspect an increase in skin cancers to be probable in future years from the widespread and, in my opinion, ill-advised use of preparations containing 5-*

methoxypsoralen. My concern is not helped by the knowledge
that DNA repair mechanisms may be less than optimal in,
perhaps, one person in 100.

Sunscreens have been known to cause allergies, and a combination of sunscreen and sunlight can trigger photosensitivity in susceptible individuals. But perhaps the most important thing to bear in mind is that sunscreens are designed to protect against sunburn: there is no scientific proof that they are effective in preventing basal cell carcinoma or, for that matter, malignant melanoma. Aside from skin cancer there is also the problem of premature ageing caused by the sun's rays. Sunscreen products are now widely promoted as having anti-ageing properties. Given the obsession with youth and a youthful self-image which permeates all of western culture, it is not surprising that sunscreen manufacturers are advocating routine everyday use of sunscreen lotions and moisturizers with UV protection. But rather than relying on blocking agents and lotions, anyone concerned about sunlight causing premature ageing may have more to gain from adopting a diet which protects against damage from the sun and wearing a hat.

SUNLIGHT, FREE RADICALS AND VITAMINS

The physicians who used sunlight as a medicine during the first half of the 20th century were well aware of the influence of diet on the recovery of their patients. Nourishing meals were an integral part of the treatment; and it seems reasonable to suggest that well-nourished skin responds better to sunlight than skin that is low in minerals. Certainly there is evidence to support the view that many of our current problems with sunlight, skin cancer and premature ageing stem from the deficiencies of our highly refined western diet.

When sunlight burns it excites free radicals in the skin. Free radicals are highly reactive molecular fragments that can combine very destructively with other molecules in the body, in a process called oxidation. They are formed in a variety of ways besides exposure to the sun: as by-products of normal metabolic processes, from cigarette smoke, alcohol consumption, and environmental pollution. Free radical reactions cause damage to cells — including their genetic material (DNA) — and are linked with a wide range of diseases including cancer, heart disease, arthritis and the ageing process itself.

Many of the latest sunscreens contain antioxidants which are supposed to neutralize any sun damage as it happens in the skin. However, vitamins A, B, C and E in the diet, together with selenium, bioflavinoids, beta-carotene (a precursor of vitamin A in the body), zinc and a number of other minerals and compounds are known to be capable of either preventing free radicals from forming, or protecting the body from damage once free radicals have formed. Vitamin A has been used to treat skin malignancies, and epidemiological studies suggest that vitamins A, C and E protect against some cancers.

A recent assessment of the effects of taking vitamins in the *Journal of the American Academy of Dermatology* in 1998, has shown that 2 grammes of vitamin C combined with 1,000 IU of vitamin E provides a protective effect against sunburn. In addition, beta-carotene in the diet is supposed to be particularly good at preventing free radical formation in the skin which, in turn, delays the onset of burning. Moreover, beta-carotene is known to have anti-cancer properties, so if you are going to travel to a sunny destination for your holiday, there is a good argument for taking a beta-carotene supplement in the weeks beforehand, and other vitamins while you are there. However, if you have to go out in strong sunshine for long periods when you are on holiday — because you play a sport, or ski, or sail, for example — then a high-factor sunblock on those areas of skin not covered by your clothing might be advisable: preferably one with physical protection rather than a chemically active ingredient.

The antioxidant vitamins and nutrients that inhibit free radicals excited by sunburn are also thought to prevent the formation of cataracts. Until quite recently the conventional view of senile cataract was that it was the result of an irreversible process, and it was left to reach an advanced stage at which point surgeons stepped in to replace the damaged lens. Evidence that nutrition can affect the development of cataract has been slowly building up over the past seventy years or so, to the extent that medical supplementation with antioxidants such as vitamins C and E and beta-carotene is now recommended as a preventive measure for the condition. If cataracts are caught in the early stages these and other antioxidants can be used to reverse some of the damage already done. This is good news for those who may be at risk of developing the condition, such as diabetics, women exposed to German measles during pregnancy, heavy smokers and drinkers, and people with chronic kidney or heart problems.

The subject of nutrition is addressed in more detail in chapter 5 but, to return to the merits or otherwise of sunscreens, there are other disadvantages to using them beyond those already discussed. As sunscreens inhibit the natural protective response of the skin to sunlight, they would be a hindrance rather than a help to anyone practising sunlight therapy, making it very difficult to monitor the natural progression of the tanning process, or the response of patients to sunlight. The physicians who used sunlight to treat tuberculosis and war wounds achieved their cures by exposing their patients gradually over many weeks to the full spectrum of the sun's rays, and slowly building up the skin's natural protection to the sun. If their tuberculosis patients didn't tan, then they didn't get better. They certainly were not allowed to burn in the way that people who spend fifty weeks of the year in the office and a fortnight at a Mediterranean resort are at risk of doing. Indeed, one of the problems with sun tanning products is that they encourage people with this sort of lifestyle to try to get a tan when they should not be in strong sunlight at all.

3

How Sunlight
can Prevent
Serious Health Problems

Each year lack of sunlight probably kills many thousands more people in this country and others at similar latitudes than skin cancer. At first glance this may seem a rather outrageous statement but it could be true. In 1995 almost 1400 men and women in England and Wales died of malignant melanoma. Coronary heart disease killed 139,000 of their compatriots in the same year. Clearly, if sunlight had only a small protective effect against heart disease then the number of lives saved by regular moderate exposure to the sun would greatly outweigh the number lost to malignant melanoma. The same argument can be applied to a number of other serious degenerative and infectious diseases that together claim hundreds of thousands of lives in Britain each year, and which appear to be associated with sunlight deprivation.

The diseases discussed in this chapter are thought by some researchers to be linked to inadequate levels of vitamin D in the body. What you have to bear in mind when you scan the table below is that in many cases the association with lack of vitamin D and sunlight has not been proven, but this is largely due to the fact that, until quite recently, comparatively little research has been carried out into the effects of vitamin D on the immune system. Another thing to bear in mind is that in Britain, as elsewhere, the vitamin D status of the general population has not been measured. So we could all have rather less of it circulating in our bloodstream than we need to have. Before we start looking at specific diseases, perhaps it would be as well to try and determine how prevalent vitamin D deficiency, or insufficiency, really is by looking at the results of some of the latest research on the subject.

Table 2: Lack of sunlight, and diseases related to it
Breast cancer
Colon cancer
Diabetes
Elevated blood pressure
Heart disease
Multiple sclerosis
Ovarian cancer
Osteomalacia
Osteoporosis
Prostate cancer
Psoriasis
Rickets
Seasonal Affective Disorder
Tooth decay
Tuberculosis

HOW COMMON IS VITAMIN D DEFICIENCY?

There seems little doubt that throughout much of northern Europe and the United States vitamin D deficiency is a very common problem among elderly people. A recent European study showed that in the winter months more than a third of 70-year-olds are deficient. According to a paper published in the *Lancet* in 1995, scientists measuring levels of vitamin D in the blood of 824 elderly subjects in 11 European countries found that levels in 36 per cent of men and nearly half the women were deficient. Those who took oral supplements or exposed themselves to UV radiation from sunlamps had satisfactory levels but, surprisingly, the lowest levels were found in the warmer southern European countries. Further investigation showed that wearing clothes to protect from the sun — the normal custom — was a strong predictor of vitamin D deficiency. The elderly are often house bound or confined to nursing homes and are unable to get into the sun. So, if they do not take vitamin D to compensate for lack of sunlight, and their diets are lacking in calcium, they are at considerable risk from fractures and bone disorders. As far as oral supplements are concerned, some of the latest research suggests that in the absence of sunlight the elderly may need as much as 800 IU of vitamin D a day, and this level of supplementation may be required after only a few weeks spent indoors. This is enough time for the effects of sunlight deprivation to become apparent if you have not built up reserves of vitamin D to cope with it.

Vitamin D deficiency is not restricted to the house bound elderly. A study of young men on normal diets who were deprived of sunlight by being kept indoors at the Royal Navy's Institute of Naval Medicine, showed that within six weeks their vitamin D stores had fallen sufficiently to cause inadequate absorption of calcium and a negative calcium balance. After two months of this regime their vitamin D levels had fallen by half and they had begun to lose calcium at a faster rate than they could take it in. By the tenth week there was a shortfall of one third in the calcium intake they needed to maintain a healthy balance. So, the prospects for anyone on a normal diet who is housebound or institutionalized are not favourable if they are unable to get out into the sun. Patients who have been in hospital for several weeks are clearly at risk. As Dr Damien Downing suggests in his book *Day Light Robbery*, if you are having bone surgery, try not to spend too long in hospital beforehand as a deficiency of vitamin D might well prejudice your chances of a speedy recovery. Fifty years ago, it was common for orthopaedic patients to be wheeled outside in their beds in good weather so that they could derive some benefit from any sunlight and fresh air that was available. While they were outside braving the elements, nursing staff could ensure the wards were thoroughly ventilated and cleaned. Needless to say, modern hospitals are no longer designed for this. If the extent of vitamin D deficiency amongst hospital patients is as significant as some studies suggest, there are grounds for architectural modifications.

Having looked at the vitamin D status of the elderly and institutionalized, what about the wider populations of northern industrialized nations? Is vitamin D deficiency as common amongst otherwise healthy adults in the general population as it appears to be amongst the elderly? The latest findings suggest that the problem may be far more widespread in developed countries than it once appeared to be. Researchers at Boston's Massachusetts General Hospital recently found that 66 per cent of patients on a general medical ward who consumed less than the recommended daily amount of vitamin D were deficient. These patients were younger than those in many earlier studies of vitamin D status, with an average age of 62 years, and only a minority of them were housebound or residents of a nursing home before being admitted, so they could be considered to be broadly representative of the general population.

What is particularly striking about the findings of this research, which was published in the *New England Journal of Medicine* in 1998, is that low levels were found in 46 per cent of patients taking multivitamins, many of which contained 400 IU of vitamin D. Of the patients who had actually consumed more than the recommended daily allowance of vitamin D for their age, one in three were still deficient. One possible explanation for this shortfall is that when the recommended daily intakes were calculated for the citizens of the United States it was assumed that everyone would be getting a proportion of their vitamin D from the sun. Hospital patients, as we have already seen, are not well placed to do this. But if the general population in urban areas in the United States are not taking the recommended amount and are not getting out in the sun either, then it is reasonable to conclude that the prevalence of vitamin D insufficiency, if not deficiency, is rather high.

The problem is not confined to the United States. The results of a survey of the vitamin D status of adults living in cities throughout France published in the journal *Osteoporosis International* in 1998 confirms that there is a high prevalence of insufficiency amongst the adult populations in urban areas because they lack sunlight exposure. Dairy products are not fortified with vitamin D in France, and the average daily intake is usually less than 100 IU a day, so vitamin D status depends mainly on the amount of sunlight available. In this study the lowest levels of vitamin D were measured in the north and centre of the country and the highest in the south west.

SUNLIGHT AND BRITTLE BONES

The incidence of hip fracture shows a similar geographical distribution to vitamin D insufficiency in France, being higher in the east and centre of the country than in the sunny west and south. This is significant, because if there were a major problem with vitamin D status amongst a large section of the urban populations of developed countries, then one might reasonably expect to see a correspondingly high incidence of degenerative bone disease and hip fractures. Traditionally, sunlight deprivation has been linked with weak or brittle bones. One of the earliest references to this was made more than two thousand years ago by the Greek historian Herodotus (480–425 BC), who noted a marked difference between the remains of the Egyptian and Persian casualties at the site of battle of Pelusium which took place in 525 BC:

'At the place where this battle was fought I saw a very odd thing, which the natives had told me about. The bones still lay there, those of the Persian dead separate from those of the Egyptian, just as they were originally divided, and I noticed that the skulls of the Persians were so thin that the merest touch with a pebble will pierce them, but those of the Egyptians, on the other hand, are so tough that it is hardly possible to break them with a blow from a stone. I was told, very credibly, that the reason was that the Egyptians shave their heads from childhood, so that the bone of the skull is indurated by the action of the sun — this is why they hardly ever go bald, baldness being rarer in Egypt than anywhere else. This, then, explains the thickness of their skulls; and the thinness of the Persian's skulls rests upon a similar principle: namely that they have always worn felt skull-caps, to guard their heads from the sun.

Herodotus, 'The Histories'

OSTEOPOROSIS, THE 'SILENT EPIDEMIC'

The bone disease osteoporosis is becoming so common in western countries as to be termed a 'silent epidemic'. Osteoporosis affects one in three women over fifty in the UK and one in twelve men. Each year about 50,000 wrist fractures, 40,000 vertebral fractures and 60,000 hip fractures are diagnosed annually. Some 20 per cent of these hip fractures are followed by death, and those who survive often suffer permanent disability and dependency. More women die as a result of hip fractures than cancer of the cervix, ovary and womb combined. For reasons that are not fully understood, bone quality is deteriorating amongst a significant proportion of the older population, and low levels of vitamin D are implicated.

Typically, women begin to lose about one per cent of their bone mass each year from about the age of 30 to 35, and men from the age of about 55. When women reach the menopause this loss can accelerate because oestrogen, which helps their bones to absorb calcium, begins to decline. In some individuals bones become thin and honeycombed, and are prone to fractures which can occur spontaneously. The hip and wrist are most susceptible, and crumbling of the spine is common. Loss of height and spinal deformity — the so-called 'Dowagers Hump' — characterize the disease. Injuries caused by osteoporosis can be very difficult to cure, as by the time the disease is diagnosed or a fracture occurs the structure of the bone has altered to such an extent that as much as a third of bone mass may have been lost. The orthodox view is that the condition is largely irreversible, so treatment is aimed at preventing further bone loss, rather than rebuilding the remaining skeleton.

In men, osteoporosis can be caused by low levels of the hormone testosterone or other health problems, but nearly half the cases of male osteoporosis has no known cause. Where women are concerned, hormone replacement therapy is considered the most effective way to halt the decrease in bone mass which occurs after the menopause. Osteoporosis may have more to do with a weakened immune system or poor nutrition than hormonal imbalance. With advancing age the intestine becomes less efficient at absorbing calcium from the diet, and the British diet probably contains insufficient calcium to compensate for any persistent loss from the body. But, whatever the cause of osteoporosis, the disease places a tremendous strain on public resources because of the cost of operations and aftercare. In the UK, the National Health Service spends more than £900 million on the treatment of osteoporosis each year. With the populations of western countries ageing, osteoporosis seems likely to place an ever increasing burden on already overstretched healthcare systems. More than one million skeletal fractures occur annually in the United States as a result of osteoporosis, of which 300,000 are hip fractures. The World Health Organization estimate that worldwide the annual number of hip fractures could rise from 1.7 million in 1990 to 6.3 million by 2050.

At the present time, conventional medical thinking holds that lack of sunlight does not play a major role in the genesis of the disease. This is understandable given the current attitudes towards the sun, and the fact that no one seems to have examined to any great extent the relationship between osteoporosis and sunlight exposure. But lack of sunlight does seem to exacerbate the disease. It has been recognized for over two decades that vitamin D deficiency is associated with increased risk of hip fracture: some studies suggest that roughly 30 to 40 per cent of elderly patients with hip fractures are deficient or insufficient. More significantly, there is a pronounced seasonal variation both in bone density and in the incidence of hip fractures. Bone density is at its lowest during the winter, more hip fractures occur in the winter months than at other times of the year, and hip fractures become more common with increasing latitude. Most falls and fall-related injuries take place in the home, so this seasonal variation in fractures is not due to ice and snow causing falls.

There is evidence that the over seventies can benefit from taking calcium and vitamin D supplements. A study published in the *Lancet* in 1994 showed that women in homes for the elderly who received a daily dose of 800 IU of vitamin D and 1200 mg of calcium over an 18-month period had a reduced risk of fracture. Some 3,270 women took part, and there was a 25 per cent reduction in the number of fractures after three years of treatment compared to those women who did not receive the supplements. There have since been other studies which show that non-vertebral fractures in the elderly can be reduced by giving oral vitamin D and calcium supplements, but the relative contribution of vitamin D and calcium is not known.

While it is much more convenient for the elderly to take supplements rather than sunbathe, this dietary approach to the problem means that they are denied all of the other benefits that sunlight exposure could bring besides the synthesis of vitamin D in the skin. Of course, like modern hospitals, elderly people's homes are not designed for sunbathing. The days of sun lounges, verandahs and porches are long gone, as is the solarium. In view of the osteoporosis epidemic, and the incidence of other degenerative diseases which may be linked to sunlight deprivation, designers should be encouraged to include them. Alternatively, sunlamps could be introduced as it is established that ultraviolet radiation from artificial sources will correct vitamin D deficiency in the elderly. However, given current concerns about skin cancer, ultraviolet radiation is unlikely to be adopted in favour of oral supplements for the foreseeable future.

As far as osteoporosis is concerned the conventional view is that the best way to prevent it in later life is to build up high bone mass during childhood and adolescence by taking regular exercise and getting plenty of vitamin D and calcium. Then, if calcium has been absorbed to a sufficient degree, the loss of bone mass associated with ageing starts from a level that is less likely to drop below the 'fracture threshold', at which point the risk of breaking bones increases. In practice, this means either getting out in the sun or taking oral supplements such as cod-liver oil, and engaging in strenuous activities during childhood. Yet parents are currently being actively discouraged from exposing infants to sunlight, and are being advised to put factor 15 sunscreen on their children whenever they go outside in the summer months. This may prevent sunburn, but not bone disorders in later life.

RICKETS AND OSTEOMALACIA — THE 'DISEASES OF DARKNESS'

There are several diseases which are traditionally associated with sunlight deprivation but the most widely known is called rickets. This used to be a very common condition in this country and, although medical textbooks refer to rickets as a dietary-deficiency disease caused by a lack of vitamin D, it was actually caused by air-pollution blocking out the sun's ultraviolet rays.

During the 17th and 18th centuries the bulk of the urban population in Europe and North America lived in overcrowded insanitary slums, with narrow, sunless alleyways and dark courtyards. As the Industrial Revolution got under way, and in the years that followed, these slums were covered in a permanent pall of smoke produced by the burning of coal in homes and factories. One of the constituents of this smog was sulphur dioxide, a gas which causes respiratory problems and acid rain. Sulphate particles can also form a persistent layer of acid haze which reflects ultraviolet radiation at the very wavelengths that are needed to synthesize vitamin D in the skin. So, thanks to a combination of bad housing and air pollution there were few opportunities for children to get enough sunshine. Not surprisingly, rickets was endemic at this time and became known as the 'English Disease'.

Children living in these inner-city areas who had severe rickets suffered from bone deformities and muscle weakness. Their bones softened with the result that there was an outward curvature of their legs and a curvature of the spine. Their teeth were late coming through and often fell out. This softening, weakening and demineralisation of the bones also affected adults, in whom the condition is referred to as osteomalacia. Although rickets was rarely fatal in itself, it resulted in high rates of infant and maternal deaths: women who had developed the disease in childhood often had deformities of the pelvis which made childbirth very hazardous.

At the beginning of the 20th century there were towns and cities in which more than 80 per cent of the children were affected by rickets, irrespective of social class, and there was still a great deal of confusion as to the cause. Some said it was lack of exercise; others that it was an infectious disease. Two other popular theories were that it was the result of a poor diet, or that it was caused by lack of fresh air and sunlight. Research into the causes of the disease followed two distinct paths. In 1918, scientists discovered that rickets could be cured in animals by feeding them cod-liver oil, which contains high levels of vitamin D. Having shown that vitamin D could cure rickets, it was assumed that it was a disease caused by vitamin deficiency; and subsequent studies by nutritionists reinforced the view that diet and vitamin D were the most important factors. Yet, at the same time, it finally became clear to scientists and physicians that rickets develops when people are deprived of sunlight, a fact which had largely been ignored in spite of strong scientific and circumstantial evidence.

Although it was known that sunlight could cure or prevent this crippling bone disease, few physicians in the 19th century were prepared to accept that something so simple as sunbathing could be an effective remedy. Indeed, to this day, it is still widely held that rickets is a disease of bad diet rather than lack of sunlight. Contrary to popular belief, and much conventional medical thinking, rickets and osteomalacia are diseases of darkness and not diet. Providing you get sufficient exposure to the sun, a diet lacking in vitamin D will not cause these diseases.

TUBERCULOSIS AND THE SUN

Moving from a country which has many hours of sunshine each day to one where sunlight is in relatively short supply can lead to vitamin D deficiency. In Asian families, infants who are breast-fed for long periods are prone to vitamin D deficiency, rickets, if their mothers are not getting sunlight or taking vitamin supplements. Women who come to Britain from South Asia are particularly susceptible to tuberculosis because their diet, strict dress codes and tendency to remain indoors prevent them getting sufficient sunlight and vitamin D to ward off the disease. In their country of origin, where sunlight is strong, the small areas of skin they expose to the sun when wearing traditional clothes are adequate for the photochemical production of enough vitamin D to stay healthy. But not in Britain, where the sun shines far less often and its ultraviolet rays are weaker. So, their vitamin D levels can fall rapidly in the first year after their arrival, and the risk of their developing active tuberculosis then remains high for the first five years of residence. Elderly white males are also sometimes at risk of developing TB because they show the same tendency to remain indoors during the day and consume a diet which lacks vitamin D.

Tuberculosis is a disease which was once thought to have been vanquished but which has moved back to the top of the public health agenda during the last decade. The incidence of tuberculosis in the UK population peaked in the early 1800s and then fell steadily as public health reforms were introduced and nutrition, hygiene and housing improved. At one time the so-called 'white plague' killed more of the UK population than all other infectious diseases combined, but by the 1950s, when drugs such as streptomycin became available and the BCG vaccination was introduced, tuberculosis was no longer the threat to public health it once had been.

With the apparent defeat of TB in the UK and in other developed countries in the years that followed, pharmaceutical companies saw little merit in developing new drugs, so fundamental scientific research into the disease came to a halt and has only recently resumed. Fifty years after the introduction of streptomycin, tuberculosis is still responsible for more deaths worldwide than any other single infectious disease. Some eight million people contract tuberculosis each year and three million die from it. The incidence of the disease is increasing in both developing and industrialized countries, partly because of the emergence of strains that are resistant to the limited range of available antibiotics. These strains are becoming established in the developed world and elsewhere, posing a serious threat to international public health.

Tuberculosis requires treatment with a combination of antibiotics for anything from six months to over a year. Any interruption in the programme allows the bacterium to develop resistance to the drugs and, as a consequence, become more dangerous. In the UK tuberculosis is still comparatively rare: there are now about 6,500 new cases each year. About 5 per cent of these new cases are resistant to one antibiotic, and just over 1 per cent are multi-drug resistant. Tuberculosis has close associations with the human immunodeficiency virus (HIV) which causes AIDS. The chances of someone infected with tuberculosis going on to develop the active form of the disease are much higher if they are also carrying HIV infection: they succumb as their immune system deteriorates. In several parts of the Third World these two diseases, tuberculosis and AIDS, have been spreading concurrently, with tragic consequences.

About a third of the world's population is infected with tuberculosis bacteria. But in the vast majority of cases the body's immune system keeps the bacteria dormant or inactive. This is because when the bacteria enter the body via the respiratory system they become enclosed in the lymph nodes around the lungs where they are coated in layers of calcium. These enclosures can break down. Poor general health, poor immune status, malnutrition, alcoholism and drug abuse can cause this to happen, but most infected people lead normal healthy lives and only 5 to 10 per cent develop active tuberculosis.

The symptoms of tuberculosis include a cough, rapid loss of weight, loss of appetite, night sweats and haemoptysis — spitting blood when coughing. Tuberculosis is usually diagnosed after a chest X-ray has been taken and a sample of phlegm examined under a microscope. Patients who have bacteria visible in their sputum are usually admitted to hospital. After a minimum of a fortnight's treatment they are non-infectious and can continue their drug therapy at home. In cases where the disease has reached an advanced stage, patients may have to spend long spells in special wards. The microbe *Mycobacterium tuberculosis* is carried from one person to another in airborne droplets, so it can be spread by coughing and sneezing. It can also be spread by spitting, and can attach itself to dust particles. Given the right conditions, tuberculosis bacteria can stay viable for months; but fortunately it is quite difficult to become infected unless one is in a confined space with little fresh air circulating and no sunlight. This is why tuberculosis often spreads amongst poorer families who live in cramped conditions, or homeless people in crowded, badly ventilated public dormitories, or amongst inmates in overcrowded prisons.

'SURGICAL TUBERCULOSIS'

Sunlight can help prevent tuberculosis developing in susceptible individuals by keeping up their vitamin D levels, and it can also prevent the disease spreading in dwellings by killing the bacterium. This is why there has been such a close association between sunlight and tuberculosis in the past. The beneficial effects of sunlight on tuberculosis patients were widely recognised in the early years of the 20th century. Sunlight therapy was used to prevent people who were susceptible to the disease from developing it, and also to spare those who had tuberculosis from the attentions of surgeons.

The most common form of the disease is tuberculosis of the lungs, or pulmonary tuberculosis. There are other forms which can manifest in the joints, bones, spine, intestines and skin. These are now referred to collectively as extra-pulmonary tuberculosis, but used to be called 'surgical tuberculosis'. This is because during the second half of the 19th century, with the introduction of anaesthetics and antiseptics, surgery had entered what was to become known as its 'golden era', and radical, intensive surgery became the accepted treatment for non-pulmonary forms of the disease. The results of all this surgical activity were often disappointing: patients were left permanently disfigured or crippled, with no guarantee that the tuberculosis would not return. So rather than resort to surgery, some physicians began to use so-called 'conservative' measures such as nutritional therapy, exercise and fresh air to improve their patients' general health, and increase their resistance to the disease. A few used sunlight. And so it was a revolt against surgery which brought heliotherapy back from obscurity and into mainstream medical practice, as we shall see in Chapter 4. Given the right conditions, the sun's rays can be used to prevent and treat tuberculosis. They may also have rather more positive influence on other diseases, such as cancer, than is generally accepted.

SUNLIGHT AND CANCER PREVENTION

Vitamin D performs a number of important functions besides its role in mineral absorption. By regulating the level of calcium in the blood Vitamin D influences the nervous system, as calcium aids nerve impulse transmission and muscle contraction. It influences the secretion of insulin by the pancreas and plays an important part in regulating the body's immune system. Vitamin D is also involved in the growth and maturation of cells: in laboratory experiments the biologically active form of vitamin D has been shown to inhibit the growth of cancer cells.

Skin cancer, in all its forms, is much more common than it used to be. In Nordic countries the incidence of malignant melanoma is increasing by an average of 30 per cent every five years, and there are now over 100,000 new cases worldwide each year. As a result of the rapid increase in skin cancer in Europe, Scandinavia, North America and Australasia there are now annual public health campaigns which advocate avoidance of the sun. What tends to be overlooked in these campaigns is that skin cancer is only one of a number of cancers that are on the increase. Cancer is now the cause of a quarter of all deaths in the UK, and claims about 146,000 lives each year. It is the most common cause of mortality after coronary heart disease, with some 300,000 new cases registered annually.

In 1911, about 7 per cent of the UK population, some 37,000 in total, died of cancer each year. By 1980 it was generally held that one in four people would develop cancer over the course of their lives and one in five would die from it. Now we are told that one in three of us are destined to develop the disease and, in a recent study commissioned by the charity Macmillan Cancer Relief, it was predicted that cancer will affect one in two Britons in the next generation. Much of the steady increase in the incidence of cancer during the 20th century is attributable to smoking, but not all. The Macmillan study forecasts that prostate cancer will triple by 2018 with more than one in four men affected during their lifetime compared with one in ten in 1990. Breast cancer will rise from 9 per cent of women in 1990 to 13.7 per cent. The increase in these cancers is due, in part, to the growing proportion of elderly people amongst the population, but by no means all of these cancers can be attributed to ageing.

In some respects cancer is to industrialized countries today what tuberculosis was to the 18th and 19th century: a major cause of death and misery which defeats the best efforts of conventional medicine. Rather ironically the way cancer has been, and continues to be, managed is very similar to the way 'surgical tuberculosis' was dealt with a century ago — before heliotherapy was rediscovered. Then, as now, all of the emphasis was on removing the manifestation of the disease and not on enhancing the patient's ability to overcome it. The cure for cancer remains elusive despite the fact that billions have been spent on research over the last thirty years. Indeed, there can be few areas of scientific research that have had more resources thrown at it and have yielded such modest results. Although from time to time there are well-publicized breakthroughs in laboratory-based cancer research, the benefits to cancer patients are not clear cut.

As far as conventional medicine is concerned, the preferred methods treating cancer are surgery, radiation or chemotherapy. Cancer cells are removed or destroyed and no attempt is made to eliminate the disease by strengthening the body's natural defence systems. Indeed, chemotherapy and radiation do exactly the opposite. Against this background it is understandable that people are turning to non-interventionist 'conservative' techniques as an alternative, or supplement, to surgical and chemical remedies. A number of alternative therapies have been developed for cancer which claim to use the body's own healing powers rather than drugs or machine-medicine, with varying degrees of success. Sunlight has been used to treat cancer and there is evidence that goes back over half a century which suggests that sunlight exposure prevents deep-seated cancers from developing.

Now, although sunlight can cause basal cell and squamous cell skin cancers in susceptible people, there is a very good correlation between sunlight exposure and low incidence of internal cancers. Death rates from cancer increase with distance from the equator. Or, to put it another way, the nearer you live to the equator the less chance you have of developing an internal cancer. This association has been clearly demonstrated in a number of studies such as the one carried out in 1941 in the United States by Dr Frank Apperly. He examined the statistics on cancer deaths across North America and Canada and found that compared with cities between 10 and 30 degrees latitude, cities between 30 and 40 degrees latitude averaged 85 per cent higher overall cancer death rates; cities between 40 and 50 degrees latitude averaged 118 per cent higher cancer death rates, and cities between 50 and 60 degrees latitude averaged 150 per cent higher cancer death rates. Dr Apperly also looked at the relationship between sunlight, ambient temperature and skin cancer. He concluded that sunlight produces an immunity to cancer in general and, in places where the mean temperature is less than about 5.5°C, or 42°F, even to skin cancer. However, at mean temperatures higher than this, solar radiation causes more skin cancer despite the increased general immunity to the disease.

So, the nearer one is to the equator, the less chance there is of developing cancer of the breast, colon, lung, etc. There is an increased risk of developing skin cancer but this decreases in cooler climates with mean temperatures below 5.5°C, or 42°F. Dr Apperly appears to have been the first scientist to investigate the relationship between ambient temperature and skin cancer. He also suggested, as others have done before and since, that exposure to sunlight might be an effective way to reduce the number of deaths from internal cancers. He concluded his review of the statistics as follows:

> A closer study of the action of solar radiation on the body might well reveal the nature of cancer immunity.

There have been a number of scientific studies in the last 20 years which support the view that sunlight can inhibit cancer, and it is clear that the mortality and incidence of breast cancer and colon cancer in North America and other areas of the world increases with increasing latitude. In 1992, Dr Gordon Ainsleigh published a paper in the journal *Preventive Medicine* in which he reviewed 50 years worth of medical literature on cancer and the sun. He concluded that the benefits of regular sun exposure appear to outweigh by a considerable degree the risks of squamous-basal skin cancer, accelerated ageing, and melanoma. He found trends in epidemiological studies suggesting that widespread adoption of regular moderate sunbathing would result in approximately a one-third lowering of breast and colon cancer death rates in the United States. Colon cancer and breast cancer are the second and third leading causes of cancer deaths in North America and Dr Ainsleigh estimated that about 30,000 cancer deaths would be prevented each year if moderate sunbathing on a regular basis became the norm.

The subject was reviewed again in another American paper published in 1995, entitled *Sunlight — Can It Prevent as well as Cause Cancer?* The authors were concerned that medical research was largely directed towards investigating the harmful effects of sunlight on fair-skinned individuals, and not on people with dark skin who lived in, or had emigrated to, parts of the United States where the incidence of sunlight was low. They concluded from their review that although there was no definitive proof that sunlight and vitamin D protect humans from the development and progression of carcinomas of the breast, colon or prostate, there were good grounds for questioning any broad condemnation of moderate sun light exposure. They felt that for some Americans — those with heavily pigmented skin — lack of solar radiation could be rather more of a problem than too much: that it may well contribute to the high incidence of prostate cancer in black American men and the particularly aggressive progress of cancer of the breast in black women. The final sentence of this paper is as telling, in its own way, as the one at the conclusion of Dr Apperly's paper of 1940 quoted above. The authors suggested that the:

> ... *study of the beneficial effects of sunlight on cancer*
> *progression should be removed from the realm of mysticism and*
> *thrust in to the scientific arena of experimental studies.*

Significantly, recent laboratory research confirms that vitamin D deficiency may be an important factor in the emergence of cancer of the breast as well as cancer of the colon, prostate and, to a lesser extent, leukaemia, lymphoma and melanoma. Scientists are getting to grips with the mechanisms which account for vitamin D's capacity to retard the progress of cancer. So, the findings of epidemiological studies of sunlight and cancer are supported by work in the laboratory. There are trials under way to see if the vitamin D can be used to treat prostate cancer and other malignancies. There do not, however, appear to have been any major clinical trials to establish whether sunlight can be used in cancer therapy, although there have been reports of its use.

Colon Cancer and the Sun

With health campaigns warning against sunbathing because of the risks of developing cancer it easy to see why the cancer inhibiting properties of sunlight have been largely overlooked. Certainly, there has been little support for the hypothesis that sunlight inhibits the development of internal cancers from mainstream cancer researchers. This is not altogether surprising given the slowness with which the association between rickets and sunlight came to be accepted by much of the medical establishment.

During the 18th and 19th centuries, rickets occurred mostly at latitudes of 37 degrees or higher, in towns and cities where air pollution reduced the amount of sunlight that would otherwise have been available. There are some striking parallels between rickets and cancer of the colon, in that almost all western countries at latitudes north of 37 degrees in the northern hemisphere, or south of that latitude in the southern hemisphere, have high rates of colon cancer. It is the second leading cause of death from cancer, after lung cancer, in the United Kingdom, the United States, Canada, Ireland and New Zealand and, as was the case with rickets, the problem is worse in areas with high levels of air pollution.

The first epidemiological research suggesting that vitamin D from sun exposure has a protective effect against colon cancer was published in the *International Journal of Epidemiology* in 1980 by Drs Frank and Cedric Garland (*see* Table 3). They looked at the geographic distribution of cancer deaths in the United States and found that mortality from colon cancer decreased in areas of the United States with greater sun exposure, the number of deaths in the industrialized northeast of the United States being one third higher than in sunnier regions such as Hawaii, New Mexico and Arizona. Migration to a sunny latitude — from, say, New York to Florida — is associated with a decreased risk of colon cancer. Also, a childhood and adolescence spent in one of the world's sunnier regions reduces the risk of the disease for those who migrate in the opposite direction, and the protective effect appears to last a lifetime.

BREAST CANCER AND THE SUN

Breast cancer is the most common form of cancer in women, causing about 370,000 deaths annually worldwide. Each year some 220,000 women in Europe and 180,000 women in North America are diagnosed with the disease. About 15,000 British women die of breast cancer annually, a death rate that is higher than elsewhere in western Europe. One in 12 British women will develop breast cancer at some time in their lives and, as we have already seen, the incidence of breast cancer is increasing. The reasons for this are not altogether clear, but lack of sunlight could be a factor. In 1989 the Drs Garland, together with Dr Edward Gorham, published the first ever epidemiological work on the relationship between sun exposure and breast cancer (*see* Table 4). Their research demonstrated that, as in the case of colon cancer, there was a strong negative correlation between available sunlight and breast cancer death rates. The chances of women from areas of the United States with less available sunlight dying of breast cancer were 40 per cent higher than those of women who lived in Hawaii or Florida. Worldwide, the lowest rates for breast and colon cancer occur in the

Table 3: Colon Cancer and Latitude

Country	Latitude (^{0})	Death rate per 100,000 population
Northern Ireland	54	16.4
Republic of Ireland	53	16.6
England and Wales	52	15.3
Netherlands	52	14.7
Germany	51	16.5
Belgium	50	15.5
Austria	47	15.2
Switzerland	47	12.2
France	46	11.2
Canada	45	13.5
New Hampshire, USA	44	11.5
New York, USA	43	12.4
Connecticut, USA	42	11.5
Rhode Island, USA	42	12.2
Massachusetts	42	12.1
Italy	42	10.5
New Zealand	41	19.7
New Jersey, USA	40	12.9
Spain	40	7.8
Greece	39	5.2
Japan	36	9.3
New Mexico, USA	34	9.1
Arizona, USA	34	8.8
Australia	33	15.8
Israel	31	11.8
Chile	30	6.1
Florida, USA	28	9.9
Mexico	23	2.7
Hawaii, USA	20	8.5
Guatemala	15	0.5

Annual Age-Adjusted Death Rates from Colon Cancer per 100,000 Population by Latitude of Residence for Women in Selected Areas, 1986–1990. After Garland, C.F., Garland, F.C., and Gorham, E.D., 'Epidemiology of Cancer Risk and Vitamin D' in *Vitamin D: Molecular Biology, Physiology, and Clinical Applications*, (Ed. Holick, M.F.), Humana Press, New Jersey, 1999

71

Caribbean, South and Central America, North Africa and South Asia. Countries in these regions are within 20 degrees of the equator, where the sun's rays are particularly strong, and where mortality rates for breast and colon cancer are 4–6 times lower than in northern Europe or North America.

The Garlands' research shows that in the United States individuals at high risk for breast cancer also have a high risk for colon cancer. They tend to be urban, living in the less sunny and more polluted north-eastern states, where soft coal with a high sulphur content is burned extensively for electricity generation, smelting and heating. The air pollution which was responsible for their forebears developing rickets is still present. It may not be as severe, but it is still blocking out ultraviolet radiation and inhibiting the synthesis of vitamin D. This could account for the marked difference in the risk of breast and colon cancer in the urban northeast compared with rural areas. A similar association between breast and colon cancer, air pollution and latitude levels has been shown in Canada and Italy. Also, breast cancer is twice as common in the northern republics of the Soviet commonwealth — the former USSR — than in republics in the south, with intermediate rates at intermediate latitudes.

While it is clear that the mortality and incidence of breast cancer and colon cancer in North America and other areas of the world increases with distance from the equator, there is one notable exception to this trend. Japan is a heavily industrialized country which is situated at a relatively high latitude, but which has had a low incidence of breast and colon cancer. This anomaly has been attributed to the fact that the traditional Japanese diet is unusually rich in vitamin D from fish, the average intake of vitamin D there is about ten times that of the average level for adults in the United Kingdom or the United States. Dietary intake of vitamin D and calcium influences the incidence of colon cancer in a similar way to that of rickets: both vitamin D and calcium are needed to keep colon cancer and rickets at bay.

Dietary intake of fat or fibre or fruit and vegetables has very little influence on the north-south gradient of colon and breast cancer in North America. Intake of fruit and vegetables is actually slightly higher in the northeast than in the rest of the country. The consumption of high-fibre cereals and bread is lower in the south than the northeast and dietary fat intake does not vary by region across the country.

Table 4: Breast Cancer and Latitude

Country	Latitude (^{0})	Death rate per 100,000 population
Northern Ireland	54	26.9
Republic of Ireland	53	25.7
England and Wales	52	29.0
Netherlands	52	25.8
Germany	51	21.9
Belgium	50	25.6
Austria	47	22.0
Switzerland	47	24.9
France	46	19.0
Canada	45	23.5
New Hampshire, USA	44	25.0
New York, USA	43	25.6
Connecticut, USA	42	23.6
Rhode Island, USA	42	25.7
Massachusetts	42	25.0
Italy	42	20.4
New Zealand	41	25.0
New Jersey, USA	40	25.8
Spain	40	15.0
Greece	39	15.1
Japan	36	5.8
New Mexico, USA	34	19.4
Arizona, USA	34	20.0
Australia	33	20.5
Israel	31	22.5
Chile	30	12.7
Florida, USA	28	20.9
Mexico	23	6.3
Hawaii, USA	20	15.0
Guatemala	15	2.3

Annual Age-Adjusted Death Rates from Breast Cancer per 100,000 Population by Latitude of Residence for Women in Selected Areas, 1986–1990. After Garland, C.F., Garland, F.C., and Gorham, E.D., 'Epidemiology of Cancer Risk and Vitamin D' in Vitamin D: Molecular Biology, Physiology, and Clinical Applications, (Ed. Holick, M.F.), Humana Press, New Jersey, 1999

PROSTATE CANCER AND THE SUN

Prostate cancer shows a similar geographic variation to cancers of the breast and colon. The known risk factors for this cancer are older age, dark skin and northern latitudes, all of which are associated with a decreased synthesis of vitamin D. The highest rates of prostate cancer occur in the United States, Canada and Scandinavia, while Japan has a low incidence of the disease. A study published in the journal *Cancer* in 1992 found that there was a significant north-south trend in the United States with a reduction in deaths from the disease as sunlight intensity increased. Mortality rates were highest in the northeast of the United States and lowest in the southwest. They were also lower amongst white-skinned Americans than in African-Americans and this could not be attributed to any differences in socioeconomic status. In common with breast and colon cancer, mortality rates from prostate cancer show an inverse association with the availability of ultraviolet radiation from the sun. As prostate cancer is the most prevalent non-skin cancer amongst men in the United States, and the second leading cause of male cancer deaths, this is an illuminating piece of research for older men — especially those with darker skin who are at higher risk of developing this condition.

OVARIAN CANCER AND THE SUN

The incidence of ovarian cancer is higher in North America and northern Europe than in Africa and Asia; with some of the lowest levels in Japan. A study published in the *International Journal of Epidemiology* in 1994 showed that in the United States there is a strong inverse association between mean daily solar radiation and deaths from ovarian cancer. Women aged between 45 and 54 living in northern states were shown to have five times the ovarian cancer mortality rate of women of this age group living in the south of the country. Of course there is, as yet, no proof that sunlight prevents ovarian cancer or any other forms of internal cancer from developing. But, then again, there is evidence, albeit limited, that some cancer patients actually benefit from exposure to the sun.

SUNLIGHT THERAPY AND CANCER

There have been a number of reports of sunlight being used on cancer patients to good effect but, unfortunately, much that has been published on the subject is largely anecdotal. One form of cancer which clearly benefits from sunlight exposure is, ironically, a form of skin cancer. This is the rare malignant skin cancer *mycosis fungoides* which has been treated very successfully with the sun's rays. The results of a study carried out at a clinic in Davos, Switzerland, reported in the journal *Hautarzt* in 1986, showed that the majority of patients with this serious condition who underwent sunlight therapy in the Alps went into remission — some for over a year.

As far as internal cancers are concerned, few physicians seem to have actually used sunlight therapeutically. One notable exception is the American physician Dr Zane Kime. In his book, *Sunlight Could Save Your Life,* which was published in 1980, Dr Kime describes how he encouraged one of his patients with breast cancer to sunbathe. He took this rather unusual step following a consultation with a 41-year-old woman whose breast cancer had spread to her lungs and bones. She had already undergone a mastectomy and chemotherapy but to no avail. Dr Kime did not treat the cancer directly but, instead, introduced a programme to improve the general health of his patient. She was only allowed to eat whole foods, and all of the refined polyunsaturated oils and fats were removed from her diet. She was also encouraged to spend time sunbathing; and the combination of diet and sunlight seems to have achieved remarkable results. Within a few months the patient was back at work and in the years that followed there were no apparent symptoms of her metastasized cancer. Unfortunately Dr Kime did not devote much of his book to this episode, nor did he state how many years of remission his patient enjoyed and, sadly, Dr Kime died in 1992.

Some years before Dr Kime's apparent success, a study into the effects of sunlight on cancer was carried out at the Bellevue Medical Centre in New York. During the summer of 1959, fifteen patients diagnosed with cancer were encouraged to arrange their own sunlight therapy. They spent as much time as they could outdoors without glasses, and especially sunglasses. They were also instructed to avoid artificial light sources and television sets as much as possible. Dr John Ott, who is a renowned investigator of the effects of light on health and is probably the greatest innovator in the field since Niels Finsen, was involved in this project. It was Doctor Ott who first alerted the American public of the hazards to health posed by the emission of X-ray radiation from television sets, and he also developed some of the first full-spectrum lighting. He says in his book *Health and Light* that the results of the study of the effects of sunlight on cancer patients were sufficiently positive to justify a more detailed programme of research, but that support was not forthcoming.

The world-famous Swiss sunlight therapist Dr Auguste Rollier (1874–1954) reported some success with Hodgkin's disease, a cancer that affects the lymph glands. But when Rollier was practising heliotherapy — in the first half of the 20th century — cancer was not as common as it is today, and tuberculosis posed a much greater threat to public health. By the time cancer became a major health problem, sunlight therapy had all but disappeared from medical practice. This explains, in part, why sunlight does not appear to have been used on cancer patients to any extent.

Now although patients with Hodgkin's lymphoma seem to have benefited from Dr Rollier's sunlight therapy, in recent years several researchers have suggested that sunlight exposure actually increases the risk of developing non-Hodgkin's lymphoma, which is a different form of lymphatic cancer. Non-Hodgkin's lymphoma is one of the fastest-increasing cancers in the UK and other countries. The reasons for the rise in incidence of this cancer are not well understood, but it does occur frequently amongst people with the HIV virus, and patients whose immune systems are suppressed by chemotherapy, or by the drugs used to prevent organ rejection after transplant surgery. Individuals who are taking immuno-suppressive drugs over long periods develop cancer much more readily than the normal population. People in this position are particularly susceptible to cancers of the skin, and so must be especially careful to avoid strong sunlight. However, as far as non-Hodgkins lymphoma is concerned the most detailed research to date, published in the *British Medical Journal* in 1997, could find no positive association with sunlight. So something other than sunlight may be causing it.

SUNLIGHT AND THE HEART

The western world's number one killer is coronary heart disease. It accounts for one third of all deaths in industrialized countries annually, and 7 million deaths worldwide. If you are unfortunate enough to have a heart condition, or you come from a family with a history of heart disease, or high blood pressure, you will probably have been made aware of the impact that your lifestyle and diet can have on your future well-being. By keeping your weight down and taking regular exercise the likelihood of ill health is far less than if you pursue a sedentary way of life, eat convenience foods and smoke. As you may have gathered from chapter 1, sunlight has a marked effect on some of the imbalances in the body which are associated with heart disease. Not only does sunlight lower blood pressure and cholesterol levels, but the results of tests reported in the *American Journal of Physiology* in 1935 show that exposure to ultraviolet radiation can also increase the amount of blood ejected from the heart — the cardiac output — by as much as 39 per cent. If sunlight does influence the functioning of the cardiovascular system to anything like this extent, one would expect to see more heart disease when and where there was less available solar radiation.

More people die of heart attacks in the winter than in the rest of the year and, as with cancer, deaths from heart disease become more common with increasing distance from the equator. Blood cholesterol levels also increase with distance from the equator, and it is countries in the northwest of Europe, such as Britain, which have the highest cholesterol levels and deaths from heart disease. The highest incidence of heart disease in the British Isles is amongst less well-off families in Scotland, Northern Ireland, and the northwest of England. In a study published in the *Quarterly Journal of Medicine* in 1996, sunlight deprivation was identified as a potential risk factor. Bad housing, minimal participation in outdoor physical activities such as gardening and insufficient money for holidays in sunny places were cited as reasons for lack of sunlight exposure amongst this high-risk group.

Significantly, coronary heart disease is also particularly high amongst Indo-Asian immigrants in Britain who, as we have already seen, tend not go out in the sun. The researchers who carried out this study put forward the hypothesis that high levels of cholesterol in the blood may accelerate existing coronary heart disease but are not the cause of it. They suggest that it is a microbe — possibly the low-grade respiratory pathogen *Chlamydia pneumoniae* — which may be to blame, and that sunlight deprivation increases the opportunism of this organism in a similar manner to the way it favours tuberculosis. If this is the case, immigrants to this country who have no natural immunity to this pathogen, or whichever organism might cause coronary heart disease, would be at even more risk of infection once their immune systems become compromised due to vitamin D deficiency. Like cancer, in spite of a massive research effort, a great deal about heart disease remains unknown and unexplained. Sunlight or, rather, lack of it may have a much more significant influence on the genesis of heart disease than is currently recognized and in my opinion this needs to be thoroughly investigated as a matter of urgency.

SUNLIGHT AND DIABETES

According to the World Health Organization, approximately 135 million people suffer from diabetes mellitus worldwide. There are two main forms of the disease: insulin dependent diabetes and non-insulin dependent diabetes. The onset of insulin dependent diabetes is most common in childhood and occurs as a result of the body's auto-immune system destroying the cells in the pancreas which produce insulin. As the name implies, insulin dependent diabetes requires treatment with insulin. Non-insulin dependent diabetes is less serious and can be treated with diet, exercise, drugs which increase the production of insulin, or insulin itself. It is the more common form of the disease and accounts for almost 90 per cent of all diabetes cases. Non-insulin diabetes occurs after the age of about 40 years in people who are genetically disposed to it and who are often overweight and unfit. The World Health Organization predict that the number of people with diabetes is set to rise to 300 million by 2025 because of population ageing, unhealthy diets, obesity and a sedentary lifestyle.

A deficiency of insulin results in increased concentrations of glucose in the blood which, in turn, causes damage to blood vessels and nerves. Diabetes can lead to severe complications in the longer term, including heart attacks, kidney failure, blindness, and gangrene in the lower extremities. Heart disease kills 75 per cent of people of European origin with diabetes. Studies have shown vitamin D to have a protective effect against childhood diabetes. The results of large pan-European trial published in the journal *Diabetologica*, in 1999, suggest that vitamin D supplements taken in infancy protect against, or arrest, the initiation of a process that can lead to insulin-dependent diabetes in later childhood. If this is the case, it seems reasonable to suggest that exposure to sunlight in early childhood may be important in preventing the onset of the disease — although no one seems to have investigated this possibility.

Whether or not sunbathing can prevent insulin dependent diabetes, it is known that sunlight has a similar effect to insulin in that it lowers concentrations of glucose in the blood. As previously discussed in Chapter 1, although this is not particularly noticeable in normal individuals, the effect is dramatic in diabetics. It is for this reason that anyone who is diabetic should be careful if they sunbathe, as they may have to reduce the amount of insulin they take to maintain normal blood sugar levels if they are in strong sunlight for any length of time. As with heart disease, the incidence of diabetes is higher amongst the Indo-Asian community than the indigenous British population, and this may be another manifestation of chronic vitamin D insufficiency.

MULTIPLE SCLEROSIS

Multiple sclerosis is a disease of the central nervous system in which the myelin sheaths covering nerve fibres are damaged, leading to a range of symptoms associated with disruption of nerve function, such as paralysis and tremors. There are about 80,000 people with multiple sclerosis in the United Kingdom, and 250,000 in the USA. The cause, or causes, of the disease are not clear, but it is known that the incidence of multiple sclerosis increases dramatically with latitude, and that exposure to sunlight in childhood and adolescence protects against the disease in later life.

Latitude was first identified as an important risk factor as long ago as 1922. Then in 1960 scientists discovered that multiple sclerosis was related to the amount of sunlight available annually and during the winter months. They concluded that, directly or indirectly, solar radiation has a protective effect against the disease. There is strong circumstantial evidence that vitamin D protects against multiple sclerosis, which helps to explain why in Switzerland the disease is common at low altitudes and much rarer at high altitudes where the intensity of ultraviolet radiation is much stronger. In Norway there is a much greater prevalence of multiple sclerosis inland than on the coast, where fish is consumed in large quantities, providing an excellent source of dietary vitamin D. In other parts of the world where the diet includes large amounts of fish, such as Japan, the incidence of multiple sclerosis is lower than would be expected on the basis of latitude alone.

One explanation for the sun's role in preventing the disease is that getting sunlight into the eyes affects the immune response of the central nervous system in some, as yet unexplained, way. The authors of a recent article in the journal *Medical Hypothesis* put forward two possible explanations for this. One is that sunlight may inhibit the development of an eye condition called 'retrobulbar optic neuritis' which affects about 85 per cent of people who then go on to develop multiple sclerosis. Inflammation in the retina of the eye and in the brain is thought to be the first stage in the development of multiple sclerosis, and the sun's rays may act on the immune system to prevent this occurring. The authors also suggest that sunlight could protect against the disease in a similar way to that in which it acts to prevent another illness related to latitude, seasonal affective disorder. Bright light prevents seasonal affective disorder because, as we saw in Chapter 1, it suppresses the secretion from the pituitary gland of the neurohormone melatonin. It seems that by inhibiting the secretion of melatonin sunlight might also protect against multiple sclerosis by strengthening the immune system and preventing demyelination.

Unfortunately, over the last forty years the association of multiple sclerosis with lack of sunlight in childhood and adolescence has not been as widely recognized as it might have been. Yet, if the disease is to be avoided, irrespective of the precise mechanism involved, there are good grounds for discouraging children from wearing sunglasses, and encouraging regular moderate sunlight exposure.

SUNLIGHT AND TOOTH DECAY

Having looked at the influence of sunlight on cancer, heart disease, diabetes and multiple sclerosis, let us return to the bones or, rather, the teeth. We have to go back a long way to find published evidence of a relationship between sunlight and dental caries, but there is some. In 1939 an American study of 94,000 white males aged between twelve and fourteen years showed a clear correlation between sunlight and tooth decay. Those who lived in the northeast of the USA, where mean annual sunlight was less than 2,200 hours per year, had two thirds more cavities than their compatriots who lived in the southwest of the country and received more than 3,000 hours of sunshine per year.

The results of another investigation, published in the *Journal of Nutrition* in 1938, showed that the incidence of dental caries amongst American children varied according to the time of year. The highest incidence was found in the late winter and early spring, and very low values were recorded during the summer months. If this is correct, then there is much to be said for making routine dental appointments at the beginning of autumn when your vitamin D levels are highest and your teeth are strongest.

PSORIASIS

Sunlight therapy is particularly effective in cases of psoriasis; a benign but chronic inflammatory skin condition which affects 1-2 per cent of the World's population. The degree to which psoriasis affects sufferers can vary from a very mild form with just a few scaly red patches on the elbows, to a more severe condition where sores completely cover the body, except the face. The disease can cause significant distress and a very restricted social life, and can require hospitalization. The symptoms of psoriasis can be relieved by the administration of a photosensitizing drug, such as 8-methoxypsoralen, by mouth followed by exposure to UVA radiation. Systemic immunosuppressive drugs, such as cyclosporin, are administered in severe cases. However, heliotherapy can clear up psoriasis without the need for such strong medication. It is often preferred to conventional therapies by patients and is particularly effective in severe cases.

During the last thirty years tens of thousands of patients, mainly from western Europe, have been given sunlight therapy for psoriasis at the Dead Sea, in Israel. The high mineral content of the water, combined with solar radiation, improves the condition of about 80 per cent of the patients who go there for medical treatment. The condition has also been treated successfully with sunlight in other parts of the world. In one recent study, published in the *British Journal of Dermatology* in 1998, some 46 Finnish patients received four weeks of heliotherapy treatment in the Canary Islands, Spain. They were sent abroad because in Finland solar radiation is too weak and sunny days are too infrequent to have any real impact on long-lasting psoriasis. The study showed that it was only really cost-effective to send patients to the Canaries for the sun if their psoriasis was so severe that they required regular hospital admissions or outpatient treatments. For psoriatic patients heliotherapy remains an effective, if rather expensive, alternative to systemic drugs.

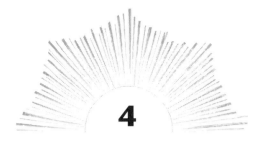

4

Sunlight:
A Medicine for Diseases
of the Past, Present and Future

The guidelines on sunbathing we are given today are much more limited than the information that was available to sunbathers half a century ago. We are told to stay out of the sun around midday, wear a hat and a T-shirt, and use high factor sunscreens, but this sort of advice is essentially negative. It tells you how to avoid sunburn but not how to make the most of sunlight's therapeutic properties. To find out how to sunbathe properly we have to learn from the past, from the days before antibiotics. So this chapter is largely concerned with the history of sunlight as a medicine.

Few doctors study the history of medicine while they are at medical school; and why should they? After all, thanks to antibiotics, over the last fifty years medical practice has changed so dramatically that they have little need to. Gone are the days when a minor cut or scratch could easily develop into fatal septicaemia, when postoperative wound infections were common, when bone infections took years to heal, and when tuberculous meningitis was invariably fatal. Now that we have effective drugs to combat these and other problems, surely there is little of any practical value to be learned from the medicine of the pre-antibiotic era?

Well, infections are becoming a major problem in hospitals. More people in Britain now die of hospital acquired infection (HAI) than are killed in road accidents. At least 5,000 people each year die as a direct result, and a further 15,000 deaths are caused by complications due to an infection caught after treatment. On average, one in 10 patients becomes infected in hospital, and at any one time one in every 10 patients is there solely because of an infection acquired after admission. It is difficult to estimate the scale of the problem because some infections do not become apparent until after patients have been discharged. Between 20–70 per cent of surgical wound infections fall into this category and such cases are not included in the statistics.

An additional problem in hospitals is that an increasing number of the bacteria that cause these infections are becoming resistant to antibiotics. Outbreaks of this kind can be very dangerous and very expensive. Infected patients have to remain in hospital for longer than those who recover normally, and the costs associated with ward closures, and the cancellation of operations and admissions runs into millions of pounds annually. In 1998, in a report on the threat to public health posed by the emergence of bacteria resistant to antibiotics, the Science and Technology Select Committee of the House of Lords reached the following conclusion:

> The evidence we have received is alarming enough as to the
> present situation, and even more so as to the prospect for the
> future. In the long term, science may come to the rescue, with
> novel antimicrobials and additional vaccines; but in the short
> term the world is facing what may be described as an epidemic
> in its own right, and the dire prospect of revisiting the pre-
> antibiotic era.

One explanation for the emergence of drug-resistant strains is the extensive use of antibiotics as feed additives for farm animals. Over 40 per cent of the antibiotics manufactured in the United States are given to animals, and in some countries antibiotics are sprayed on fruit trees to prevent or control bacterial infections. Such practices encourage the growth of resistant bacteria which, in turn, could be passed to humans whenever they eat raw or under cooked food. One of the more popular farmyard antibiotics, avoparcin, has recently been banned in Europe as a growth promoter. It is very similar in its structure to the antibiotic vancomycin, which is modern medicine's last line of defence against a range of infectious bacteria that have become resistant to all of the other drugs available. The emergence of a vancomycin-resistant strain of the enterococcus bacterium has been linked to the use of avoparcin in pigs and poultry. The salmonella bacterium could conceivably go the same way, as could a number of other pathogens.

Vancomycin-resistant enterococci are already untreatable in some hospitals around the world and another organism, the methicillin-resistant *staphylococcus aureus* (MRSA), is now a common cause of hospital infections, and is a particular danger to patients recently operated on, those with an open wound and older patients. In 1997, for the first time, three geographically separate cases infected with the *staphylococcus* microbe responded poorly to vancomycin. This was an event both anticipated and feared by doctors worldwide: it means that variants of a bacterium that causes blood poisoning, wound infections and pneumonia are upon us which are untreatable by every available antibiotic.

Resistance to drugs is thought to have been stimulated by doctors in general practice who inappropriately prescribed antibiotics for viral infections. Studies suggest that about half of the antibiotics given to patients in hospitals are incorrectly prescribed. Also, irregular use of the drugs, or failure to complete a full course of treatment, can encourage partially resistant strains to evolve into fully resistant bacteria, as we have already seen in the case of tuberculosis. What needs to be borne in mind when we are presented with the rather frightening scenario of a return to the pre-antibiotic era is that new antibiotics are being developed, and antibiotics do not constitute our main defence against infection. A high standard of hygiene, proper sanitation, a bacteriologically pure water supply, fresh air, exercise and a nutritious diet are far more important. After all, antibiotics were not responsible for the steady decline of tuberculosis in England from the 1800s onwards: this had more to do with improving living standards and public health legislation.

Another thing to bear in mind about antibiotics is that they are not without their negative effects: when they attack bacteria which cause a particular disease they also eliminate benign bacteria that might otherwise limit the growth of these pathogens, or that have an important part to play in our resistance to other infections. Furthermore, some antibiotics have significant side-effects, one of which is photosensitivity. The antibiotics tetracycline, declomycin, aureomycin and griseofulvin can render the skin more sensitive to sunlight, as can a number of other common drugs.

Antibiotic resistance is not a new phenomenon; it was apparent in the 1950s, and warnings of new plagues should be treated with a degree of caution — perhaps not as much as predictions of an epidemic of ozone-depletion-induced cancers and cataracts, but caution nevertheless. Doom and disaster sell newspapers — and books — and are good for television ratings. Predictions of global catastrophes of this kind are a great help to scientists in their constant quest to secure research money, and they enable bureaucrats to extend their influence ever wider.

However, drug resistance is a serious concern in hospitals where even the most routine surgery depends on the availability of antibiotics such as vancomycin. There is always a risk of picking up a post-operative infection from bacteria such as *staphylococcus aureus,* as a contributor to the *Journal of Tissue Viability* described in the January 1999 issue. A minor operation, followed by infection with MRSA resulted in a 9 week stay in intensive care, a heart attack, kidney failure, breathing problems and other complications. Clearly, without antibiotics to clear up an infected wound, or blood poisoning, even minor surgery could become very hazardous indeed.

Perhaps it is time to dust-off a few old medical text books and find out what doctors did in the past. One could be forgiven for thinking that they were virtually powerless to influence the course of serious infections, but this is far from the truth. The techniques they developed may be of great value to us in the years ahead if the ability of organisms to adapt and acquire resistance continues to outstrip the development of new antibiotics.

First of all we will look at the way they used cold conditions and fresh air to stimulate the body to heal itself, which became known as the 'open-air' treatment of disease; and then at the history and practice of 'heliotherapy', which is the use of sunlight as a medicine. Heliotherapy was rediscovered at the beginning of the 20th century after more than a thousand years of neglect. Its use developed from the open-air treatment of disease. So, to understand the former we have to know a little of the latter, so to speak.

But before getting too deeply involved in the finer points, there are one or two concepts to grapple with. First, each of us responds differently to sunlight. There is no rigid formula or set of rules that will result in a healthy tan and a strengthened immune system. Second, sunbathing for health is synonymous with lots of fresh air. It aim is to be invigorating. This is why so many heliotherapy clinics were either high in the mountains or on the sea shore. The way many people now sunbathe — baking in the hot sun, in warm air — should be avoided. The purpose of a healthy sun bath is to stimulate the body's defences and not to compromise them. Fresh air, sea water, or a combination of the two are the ingredients which make the difference.

The Open-Air Treatment of Infectious Diseases

If you were born much before the 1960s you may have spent a lot of time in a 'perambulator' as a baby. The chances are you were wrapped up and left outside in the pram in all weathers: snow, sleet and rain. Even if you didn't have a pram your parents would have been encouraged to expose you to fresh air and sunlight at every opportunity — to make sure you grew up to be fit and well. As a child you probably played in the street. Some of your summer holidays may well have been spent building sand castles on the beach at one of the country's coastal resorts. You probably walked or rode a bicycle to school. When you got there you will have enjoyed (or endured) a lot of outdoor games and exercises, and it is unlikely that you came home to a house that had central heating.

Things are rather different these days. There is much less emphasis on the need for children to take part in what would once have been called 'open-air' activities. This is because the childhood diseases which were common before the last war have largely disappeared. Also lifestyles have changed. For many children it is too dangerous to walk to school or play in the street and there are fewer opportunities to take part in organized sports at school than there would have been, say, twenty years ago. It is safer and easier for them to spend hours each day watching videos or playing computer games than to go outside and get some exercise. Fresh air and exercise play a much smaller role in the development of a growing child than they once did. The idea that exposure to cold fresh air could be beneficial for children was a legacy from the days before antibiotics were widely available. In the fifty years or so before drug therapy revolutionized medicine, fresh air or open-air methods as the treatment became known, together with sunlight therapy, were the mainstay in the battle against infectious diseases such as tuberculosis.

The Open-Air Treatment of Tuberculosis

For most of the 19th century throughout northern Europe and north America tuberculosis was generally regarded as hereditary, non-infectious and incurable. As it was thought that patients with the disease could not be cured, their comfort was more important than any attempt to improve their health. A warm, mild climate was considered beneficial; cold, fresh air was to be avoided at all costs. Anyone who had tuberculosis or was thought to be at risk of contracting the disease was wrapped in warm clothes and kept in a 'hothouse' atmosphere. It was fashionable to avoid draughts, while emetics and a range of noxious fumes and substances were prescribed, together with bleeding and blistering. Tuberculosis patients were sent to coastal resorts but were often confined in heated rooms and fed a meagre diet.

The first physician to criticize such practices openly was Dr George Bodington (1799–1882). He formulated the principles of the open-air treatment of the disease. He was also the proprietor of the first institution which could be described as a tuberculosis sanatorium, in Sutton Coldfield, near Birmingham.

Bodington's open-air treatment had developed from his observation that people who spent a great deal of time indoors were susceptible to tuberculosis, whilst those who worked outside, in the fresh air, were usually free of the disease:

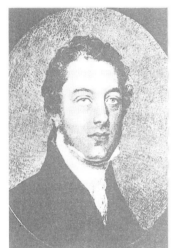

Figure 2: Dr George Bodington, the pioneer of open-air treatment of tuberculosis

Farmers, shepherds, ploughmen, etc., are rarely liable to consumption, living constantly in the open-air; whilst the inhabitants of towns, and persons living much in close rooms, or where occupations confine them many hours indoors, are its victims: the habits of the latter ought, in the treatment of the disease, to be made to resemble as much as possible those of the former class, as respects air and exercise, in order to effect a cure.

He objected strongly to the use of the popular drugs of the day, and the practice of confining patients in warm, badly ventilated rooms to protect them from the supposedly injurious effects of cold air. Bodington's patients underwent a regime of rest, diet therapy, light exercise and — above all — exposure to fresh air. He was successful in treating the disease and, in some cases, curing it. Bodington published a famous essay on the subject in 1840 at a time when, he estimated, one in five of the population of England were dying of the disease. As he put it:

Despair seems to have taken full possession of the medical profession as regards this destructive disease, and none but the feeblest efforts are exerted to oppose its progress.

The medical establishment did not take kindly to his essay, or to his methods, and he was forced to stop, but open-air treatment eventually became the accepted therapy for tuberculosis. In 1884, Edward Livingston Trudeau (1848–1915) opened one of America's first sanatoria, at Saranac Lake in New York State. The most famous German sanatorium was the Nordrach-Kolonie, in the Black Forest, which was established in 1888 by Dr Otto Walter (1853–1919). It became so well-known that 'Nordrach' became the term for open-air sanatoria; and similar institutions began to be erected throughout Europe and other countries around the world. An 'open-air recovery school' founded at Charlottenberg, a suburb of Berlin, in 1904 was the first school of its type for tubercular children, and this was copied in the same way that Germany's open-air sanatoria were. George Bodington had predicted the rise of the sanatorium in his visionary essay of 1840 and, in a letter to his son in 1866, expressed the hope that one day the pioneering work he carried out at Sutton Coldfield would receive some belated recognition:

> I often think that, when I am dead and buried, perhaps the
> profession will be more disposed to do me some justice than
> when I am alive.

So how did all of this fresh air influence the course of tuberculosis? In the 1920s scientists began to investigate open-air treatment and they discovered that what was actually happening was that cold conditions stimulated the body to produce heat and this speeded up the healing process. If exposure was carried out correctly, the body's metabolic rate (the activity of all of the body's tissue cells) increased. Research showed that this led to deeper breathing, improved circulation, increased appetite and improved digestion. In addition, the excretory and secretory glands became more active, and there was more effective removal of toxins from the tissues of the body. Of course, the idea that exposing the body to cold fresh air is beneficial goes back a long way, well before George Bodington's discovery. Hippocrates was keen on it:

> For it is not good for the body not to be exposed to the cold of
> winter, just as trees that have not felt the winter's cold can
> neither bear fruit nor themselves be vigorous… When the
> equinox has come, the days are now milder and longer, the
> nights shorter; the coming season is hot and dry, the actual
> season is nourishing and temperate. Accordingly, just as trees,

which have no intelligence, prepare for themselves growth and shade to help them in the summer, even so man, seeing that he does possess intelligence, ought to prepare an increase in flesh that is healthy.

Hippocrates, 'Regimen'

Just as gardeners put their plants out in the spring to toughen up or 'harden', so the human body seems to benefit from the stimulus of cold conditions from time to time. In fact, the term 'hardening' still appears in medical literature on climate therapy but, as you may have already gathered, opportunities to take advantage of cold fresh air in this way can be rather limited in the modern world.

SUNLIGHT THERAPY IN THE ANCIENT WORLD

Sunlight has been used as a medicine for thousands of years. The ancient Greeks used to refer to sunning the body as *heliosis*, after their sun-god Helios, and they also used to take sand baths in the sun, which they called *arenation*. The Greek physician Soranus of Ephesus (fl.110 AD) prescribed heliosis for chronic diseases including epilepsy, paralysis, haemorrhage, asthma, diseases of the oesophagus, jaundice, elephantiasis, diseases of the bladder, and obesity. He combined heliosis with various forms of hydrotherapy, such as bathing in natural springs, and sea-bathing. The Greek surgeon Antyllus, who lived about 300 AD, described sunlight therapy in his writings, as did Herodotus, a Greek physician of the second century AD.

The Romans were great believers in the healing powers of the sun's rays, and they also practised what we would now call preventive medicine. The main reason for this was that they had a mistrust of doctors, most of whom came to Rome from Greece and Asia Minor. Few Roman citizens ever became doctors as medicine was not a respectable profession. So they relied on sanitation, good water supplies, hygiene, exercise and sunbathing to keep themselves healthy. The Roman scholar Pliny the Elder (23–79 AD), who was a fierce critic of the doctors of his day, described sunbathing as *'the best of all self-administered remedies'* and used to sun himself daily, after a light lunch and before a cold bath.

The Roman philosopher Cornelius Celsus advocated exposure to the sun for the debilitated or corpulent, or those suffering from 'dropsy' (oedema). In his treatise *On Medicine,* Celsus says that swollen parts should be exposed to the sun, but not for too long in case the patient becomes feverish. The great Arabic physician and philosopher Ibn Sina, or Avicenna, (980–1037 AD) recommended sun baths for asthma and sciatica, and for the dispersion of flatulence, swellings and dropsies. In his famous *Canon of Medicine* Ibn Sina described various ways of taking sea-sand baths in the sun, including sprinkling sand over the body to remove any adverse reactions to the treatment.

With the fall of Rome and the rise of Christianity sunlight therapy fell from favour. In Rome, as in Greece, heliotherapy was closely linked with sun-worship. The early Christians had fought a long, bitter campaign against pagan solar cults and, once their church had become established, they wasted no time in killing off overt sun-worship in all its forms. Unfortunately, knowledge of the healing powers of the sun seems to have disappeared from the collective consciousness at about the same time. The Dark Ages spelt the end of sunlight therapy in Europe for over a thousand years.

THE REDISCOVERY OF SUNLIGHT AS A MEDICINE

In 1877 two British scientists, Dr Arthur Downes and Thomas Blunt, carried out a series of experiments to find out whether light had any influence, favourable or otherwise, on the development of bacteria or other organisms. They discovered it had a pronounced bactericidal effect, which they reported in the *Proceedings of the Royal Society*. In their first experiment they had placed eight test-tubes in a stand outside a southeast window for a month. The test-tubes contained Pasteur's solution; a mixture of water, sugar, ammonium and other ingredients favourable to the growth of bacteria. Four of the test-tubes were covered by thin sheet-lead, and four left uncovered for the duration of the experiment. They found that the test-tubes exposed to sunlight remained clear, while those that were covered became turbid, and when examined under a microscope were found to be full of bacteria.

Dr Downes and Mr Blunt had shown that sunlight was a potent lethal agent, even through glass. They also found that the visible spectrum, particularly the blue region, exerts a bactericidal effect. These discoveries prompted other scientists to investigate the effects of exposing bacteria to the sun's rays. In 1890, the German physicist and bacteriologist Robert Koch (1843–1910) showed that sunlight was lethal to the bacteria that caused tuberculosis, having discovered the tubercle bacillus, or *Mycobacterium tuberculosis* as it is now known, eight years previously and proved that it caused the disease. Robert Koch's work, and that of Dr Arthur Downes and Thomas Blunt, focused attention on the important part played by sunlight in the prevention of tuberculosis which, by the end of the 19th century, was becoming recognised as an infectious disease and not an hereditary one as had previously been thought.

Robert Koch was awarded the Nobel Prize for Medicine in 1905. Two years earlier the winner was another scientist with an interest in the effects of sunlight on tuberculosis, Dr Niels Finsen (1860–1904). Niels Finsen was the first physician both to use sunlight as a medicine and to investigate its effects scientifically, and he probably did more to show the importance of light to health than anyone before or since. Dr Finsen carried out some of the first research into the action of ultraviolet radiation on living organisms. He was then able to use the knowledge he had gained from these experiments to treat two previously incurable diseases: smallpox and tuberculosis of the skin.

Niels Finsen was born at Thorshavn in the Faroe Islands on December 15th 1860. He received his early training in medicine in Iceland and moved to Denmark when he was 20 to continue his studies. Three years later he had an

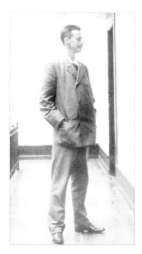

attack of rheumatic fever which seriously affected his heart and by the time he graduated from the University of Copenhagen, in 1890, he was an invalid, never to recover his health. This prevented Finsen from following a career in medicine and so he taught anatomy at the University. While studying as a medical student in Copenhagen, Finsen had noticed that he could work better in a sunny room and that he felt better out in the sun, but could find no explanation for this in his textbook of physiology. His interest in the subject grew when he watched the behaviour of a cat lying in the sun. The cat repeatedly moved into the sun every time a patch of shade reached it.

Figure 3: Dr Niels Finsen, who won the Nobel Prize for medicine in 1903, and practised sunlight therapy at his 'Light Institute' in Copenhagen

When his health would allow, Finsen's spare time was taken up investigating the effects of ultraviolet and visible radiation on living creatures and the causes of *erythema solare* — sunburn. As the name implies, it was commonly held that the heat of the sun's rays produced this effect which was referred to as 'erythema caloricum'. In 1889 Professor Erik Johan Widmark (1850–1909) of Stockholm proved scientifically that it was the sun's ultraviolet rays and not the red 'heat' rays which caused erythema and tanning of the skin. This inspired Niels Finsen to conduct a number of experiments in which he exposed himself to strong ultraviolet radiation from an electric arc-lamp. He confirmed Widmark's findings and showed that blue and violet rays can also produce inflammation of the skin, albeit to a lesser extent than ultraviolet light. It occurred to Dr Finsen that if ultraviolet radiation could produce severe inflammation of healthy skin it would do much more damage to the inflamed, sensitive skin of someone suffering from a disease such as smallpox.

SUNLIGHT AND SMALLPOX

Smallpox is a highly infectious disease, at one time endemic in many parts of the world and greatly feared because of its high mortality rate. It was called the 'speckled monster' in England because large numbers of pustules appeared on the skin of the sufferer while they were infected, and often left them permanently disfigured if they survived. In July 1893 Dr Finsen published a paper in which he put forward the theory that if smallpox patients were protected from ultraviolet radiation they would be spared the suppuration and scarring which usually characterizes this deadly disease. He had noticed that with smallpox the worst scarring occurs on the face and hands, the parts of the body most exposed to daylight. Dr Finsen reasoned that patients in the early stages of the disease needed to be kept in red light and protected from the ultraviolet 'chemical' rays of the electromagnetic spectrum. His theory was put to the test by two physicians in Norway in the same year. They found that the most dangerous and painful stage of smallpox — the period of suppuration — did not occur, and there was no swelling or temperature rise, and no pitting of the skin.

Subsequent control tests showed just how acute the sensitivity of smallpox patients to light really was. If they were exposed to the slightest amount of daylight after the beginning of his red-light treatment they would invariably suffer suppuration and scarring. In his book *Phototherapy* Niels Finsen emphasized this, as follows:

> … smallpox patients must be protected from the chemical rays with as much care as the photographer uses for his plates and paper.

Dr Finsen's 'Red-Room' therapy for smallpox was adopted by physicians in Scandinavia and Europe. Treatment had to be started as soon as the smallpox rash first appeared, before suppuration, and continue until all of the blisters on the skin had dried up. Death was not always prevented, but if the procedure was followed in good time, patients would recover with little, if any, pitting of the skin. As Niels Finsen was aware, it was a rediscovery. Similar methods had long been used as a popular remedy in China, Japan and Romania, and had been described by medieval physicians. Nevertheless, he showed that it had a scientific

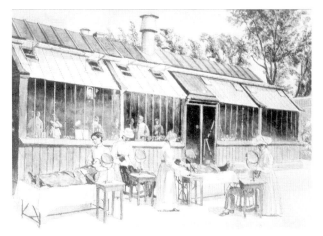

Figure 4: Patients at Finsen's 'Light Institute' being treated with ultraviolet radiation from the sun

basis and so, having established his credentials as a light therapist, Finsen turned his attention to another skin disease: *lupus vulgaris.*

Lupus was thought at one time to be cancer and was referred to as 'wolf-cancer' or 'wolf-bite' which is why it is called *lupus*, the Latin for wolf. It is a form of tuberculosis that chiefly affects the face, rarely killing directly but causing such disfigurement that death was often a relief to sufferers. The only treatment available at the turn of the century was surgery, which in many cases left patients hideously disfigured.

In 1897, Niels Finsen published a paper in which he described how he had found a cure for *lupus* using concentrated ultraviolet radiation. He found that if he focused ultraviolet rays onto the faces of *lupus* patients their tuberculosis gradually disappeared. At first he thought that this was because the ultraviolet rays were killing the TB germs but later, towards the end of his tragically short life, he felt that the ultraviolet radiation was in some way stimulating the body to heal itself.

Dr Finsen ran a 'Light Institute' in Copenhagen to which patients with *lupus vulgaris* came from around the world for his revolutionary light therapy. In summer they were treated outdoors with sunlight which was

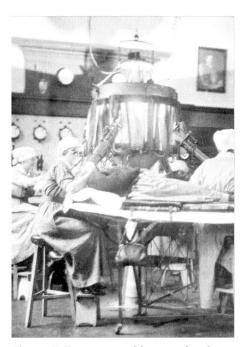

Figure 5: Treatment of lupus vulgaris with a 'Finsen Lamp'

concentrated with large magnifying lenses. In the winter he used ultraviolet radiation from specially constructed carbon-arc lamps, which became known as 'Finsen Lamps'. Although this was the work that won him the Nobel Prize in 1903, it is clear from his writing that he preferred to use sunlight, rather than light from artificial sources, when treating tuberculosis. As Niels Finsen's ideas on the healing powers of light developed he began to use electric-light baths on his patients. They lay naked, on couches, in a circular room in the middle of which were two large arc-lights suspended about six feet from the floor. Dr Finsen also encouraged patients to walk about naked in the sun, and he began to investigate the effects of sunbathing on tuberculosis of the bones, joints, skin; and on pulmonary tuberculosis. Although this work was rather overshadowed by his initial success with the Finsen Lamp, he did inspire other physicians to use sunlight to treat TB and war wounds.

WAR WOUNDS, SUNLIGHT AND OPEN AIR

Nothing in civil practice, or in previous campaigns, had prepared military surgeons for the work they had to undertake during the early years of the First World War. Wounds, particularly gunshot wounds, were far more difficult to treat than anything previously experienced. For the first time, military surgeons had to deal with the injuries caused by high-velocity weapons fired at close range. The German rifle of the period had a muzzle velocity of about 1,000 yards per second. In the first 800 yards or so, the projectile it fired 'wobbled' — the point kept steady, while the base moved round in a circle or ellipse of gradually diminishing size. On impact the bullet turned over and over, causing tearing and destruction of tissue but also leaving a zone of dead tissue around its path because of the tremendous concussion caused by the impact. At close range the momentum was such that if a bone was hit, the fragments would themselves be converted into projectiles capable of tearing into the softer tissues. In addition, mud and shreds of clothing, or pieces of flesh and bone, could be drawn into the wound. The standard issue British infantry round was, if anything, even more destructive: during the early years of the war there were complaints from the Germans that dumdum bullets were being used by the British against their soldiers.

An added hazard was that the campaign in Flanders and northern France was largely conducted on agricultural land. The fields had been heavily manured with the faecal material of horses, cows and pigs. At the start of the war British troops were often covered from head to foot with clay, earth and mud for more than a month at a time. Not surprisingly, this mud proved to be a fertile medium for micro-organisms of faecal origin such as tetanus, the gas gangrene bacillus, enterococcus and putrefactive organisms of various forms which, when carried into wounds, gave rise to highly virulent infections. This situation was compounded by the poor condition of the soldiers during the early part of the war. They were often in a state of extreme fatigue or exhaustion, which reduced their resistance to infection.

One of the methods used to try and reduce the amount of infection was to leave wounds open rather than bandage them. It was found that to bandage the wounded and send them to a base hospital for operation meant that heat and moisture, confined by the dressing, checked the production of lymph and favoured the development of gas gangrene. The laying wide open of wounds at the clearing stations at the front came to be common practice. In addition, open-air methods were adopted on a large scale for the treatment of sick and injured soldiers. As the military surgeon Lieutenant-Colonel Sir Berkley Moynihan put it in the *British Medical Journal* of March 4th, 1916:

> In the treatment of all gunshot wounds where the septic
> processes are raging, and the temperature varies through
> several degrees, an immense advantage will accrue from placing
> patients out of doors. While in France I developed a great
> affection for the tented hospitals…

Heliotherapy was also widely used to treat casualties, and hospitals were arranged for sunlight treatment. With no antibiotics, and only the most basic disinfectants, sunlight proved to be an effective agent with which to clean up wounds and speed up the healing process. Fortunately, the physician who reintroduced sunlight therapy into mainstream medical practice had discovered the beneficial effects of sunlight on wounds twelve years before the war started, and was able to bring his skills to the wounded on both sides of the conflict.

DR OSKAR BERNHARD (1861–1939): THE HEALER OF WOUNDS

Oskar Bernhard was born in Samaden, Switzerland, the son of a local chemist. He studied medicine at Zürich, Heidelberg and Berne, where he developed a particular interest in surgery. He built up a large surgical practice and helped to establish the Oberengadin District Hospital at Samaden which opened in 1898. It was here, as surgeon-in-chief, that he began to use sunlight to heal first wounds and then tuberculosis.

On the night of February 2nd, 1902, an Italian was brought to the hospital with severe knife wounds. These included a perforating wound of the chest, and two perforating wounds of the abdomen, with damage to the liver and spleen. As the injured man was in danger of bleeding to death, Bernhard had to remove the spleen, which had been pierced. Eight days later the operation wound burst open, and gaped widely, with only a few stitches holding. An attempt to re-stitch the wound failed as the edges could not be brought together again. The wound was slow to granulate (the first step in the healing process whereby red, moist tissue develops on the surface of an open wound or ulcer) and it discharged profusely. None of the treatments used to dry it up had any effect so Dr Bernhard took the unusual step, at that time, of exposing the wound to the sun:

> As I entered the hospital one beautiful morning, and the sun
> shone warmly through the open window, while a refreshing and
> stimulating atmosphere filled the whole ward, the thought
> suddenly occurred to me of exposing this large wound to the sun
> and air; for the mountain peasants of the Grisons also exposes
> fresh pieces of flesh to the sun and dry air to preserve them, and
> in this way makes a nourishing and tasty food, the well-known
> 'Bindenfleisch'. So I resolved to try this antiseptic and drying
> effect of the sunlight and air on the living tissues. Then, to the
> astonishment of the staff, I had the bed put to the open window
> and laid the large wound open. By the end of the first hour and a
> half's exposure there was a marked improvement noticeable, and
> the wound presented quite a different appearance. The
> granulations became visibly more normal and healthy, and the
> enormous wound skinned over quickly under the treatment.

> Oskar Bernhard, 'Light Treatment in Surgery'

This success led him to treat all granulating and infective wounds with sunlight. The treatment took place either in the open air on a verandah, or in the sick-ward, and the procedure was to remove the dressings and expose wounds to the sun for several hours daily. Where necessary he used a thin gauze curtain to keep off dust and flies, otherwise the wounds were unprotected. The duration of exposure was gradually lengthened, increasing every day by ten to twenty minutes up to a maximum of three to six hours, depending on the tolerance of the patient. After sunning, the wounds were left exposed to the air. At night, or at times when the wounds were not exposed to the sun, they were covered with an aseptic gauze bandage, or were protected from friction against the bedclothes by a wire cage made for the purpose. For large war wounds or large flesh wounds Dr Bernhard used wire cradles that were held in place by plaster of Paris bandages. He did not recommend sunlight for fresh uninfected wounds or primary operation wounds, which he bandaged. On the other hand he would not bandage wounds which discharged pus or sanies, the foul-smelling, thin fluid produced by a septic wound or ulcer. He explained why in his book *Light Treatment in Surgery* as follows:

> *Why should one hold up the secretion of infected wounds by thick bandages so that it may lead to great development of bacteria like an incubator? We do decidedly better with the sun and air treatment.*

Bernhard observed that, when exposed to sunlight, torpid wounds became clean and dry, the granulations smaller and fresher. Discharging ulcers and pockets which would normally have required a frequent change of dressing, and even then often continued to discharge, dried up under the treatment and the discharge of badly smelling wounds rapidly became odourless. When treating compound fractures Bernhard found that sunlight stimulated the formation of callus, the new tissue which forms around the ends of a broken bone, and that it had a marked analgesic effect.

BERNHARD'S HELIOTHERAPY OF WAR WOUNDS

During the early years of the World War I, Dr Bernhard served in German military hospitals. In the summer of 1915 he began to use heliotherapy at Bad Dürrheim in the Black Forest. At the request of the Health Department of the 14th German Army Corps he started a sun clinic in the Association Hospital at Kindersolbad for soldiers with indolent wounds, or external tuberculosis. Military sun-hospitals were then established at Dürrheim for wounded and sick soldiers from the whole German Army and the German military authorities designated Kindersolbad a 'Special Department for Radiation Treatment'.

From 1916 to 1917, Dr Bernhard acted as Swiss Military Surgeon to prisoner of war camps in Germany, England and northern France. He visited camps with the object of choosing prisoners to be sent to Switzerland for the after-treatment of wounds. During the course of his travels he saw that military surgeons were making extensive use of heliotherapy in the treatment of wounds. One hospital that he considered to be ideally arranged for heliotherapy of war wounds was the Duchess of Connaught Military Hospital which the Canadian Red Cross had built in England at Maidenhead, Berkshire, on the property of the Astor family.

DR AUGUSTE ROLLIER, THE 'HIGH PRIEST' OF SUNLIGHT THERAPY

During the Great War, Oskar Bernhard gained a reputation for conserving severely injured limbs that would normally have been amputated by other surgeons, and of never losing a patient to tetanus or gangrene. His success with sunlight brought national and international recognition, but the physician who popularized heliotherapy as a remedy for war wounds and tuberculosis was Dr Auguste Rollier (1874–1954) who began to use sunlight on his patients at a clinic in Leysin, Switzerland in 1903, one year after Bernhard. Auguste Rollier was born on October 1st, 1874, at St. Aubin in the Swiss canton of Neuchatel. He was educated at the universities of Zürich and Berne, graduating in medicine in 1898. Like Bernhard before him, Rollier studied surgery under Professor Theodor Kocher (1841–1917) at his clinic in Berne and went on to become one of Kocher's assistants. Kocher was the preeminent surgeon in Europe at this time: he was awarded the Nobel Prize in 1909 for his surgical work on the thyroid gland. Kocher's book *Operative Surgery* was the standard reference text for a generation of

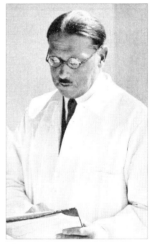

Figure 6: Dr Auguste Rollier (1874–1954) the world-famous heliotherapist

surgeons, many of whom carried out operations on children with tuberculosis. This was because children and adolescents were particularly susceptible to tuberculosis of the bones, joints and glands and, as we have already seen, the remedy generally administered was radical, intensive surgery.

To give a flavour of surgical practice at this time, in cases where tuberculosis had infected the hip, which was common in children with the disease, the joint was normally excised. This often meant removal of the head of the femur and the acetabulum — the ball and socket. Figures published in the *British Medical Journal* in 1889 show that over 36 per cent of patients died after this operation. So it is not surprising that people gradually came to the conclusion that radical surgery was not necessarily the best approach. Even after amputations tubercular children were generally far from being cured: as they were often already severely weakened by the disease, a local recurrence or a general tubercular infection often followed surgery. Rather than resort to radical surgery, some physicians at the beginning of the century began to use open-air methods and heliotherapy in an attempt to improve their patients' general health, and increase their resistance to the disease.

Oskar Bernhard, who had been treating surgical tuberculosis with open-air methods, diet therapy and orthopaedic measures from the 1880s onwards, turned to sunlight in 1902. Auguste Rollier also became disillusioned with the poor results obtained by surgery in the treatment of skeletal tuberculosis at about the same time, and two developments led him to abandon what would have been a very promising career as a surgeon. Firstly, a close friend who had contracted tuberculosis while at school with Rollier and had had his hip and knee joint excised by Kocher returned for more surgery during the period when Rollier was Kocher's assistant. Unfortunately these operations did not cure Rollier's friend of the disease and his eventual suicide left a deep impression on the young doctor. In addition, Rollier's fiancée became seriously ill with pulmonary tuberculosis so, in the hope that the high mountain air would prolong her life (which it did), Rollier left Berne and went into a rural general practice at Leysin in the Alpes Vaudoises.

It was at Leysin that Auguste Rollier pioneered a form of treatment for surgical tuberculosis in which very slow tanning in cool conditions was combined with rest, fresh air, nourishment and exercise. The aim was to strengthen his patients and improve their resistance to the disease. From the outset Dr Rollier used sun-baths rather than the local application of sunlight, as was Oskar Bernhard's practice. Auguste Rollier's method of using sunlight was copied by doctors in Switzerland, the United States and other countries around the world and, over a period of forty years, became standard procedure in a number of hospitals.

The 'Rollier Method' of heliotherapy was used on patients who were extremely sensitive to sunlight because of their weakened condition. Each individual responds to sunlight differently so the process of tanning was very closely monitored, and carefully tailored to suit each patient. Dr Rollier's methods are summarized below together with some of his findings. But first a word of caution to anyone thinking of pursuing them. Exposing anyone who is unwell to sunlight or cold air can be extremely dangerous. It takes a highly trained practitioner to be able to use solar radiation therapeutically, and it should not be attempted by anyone who is not qualified to do so.

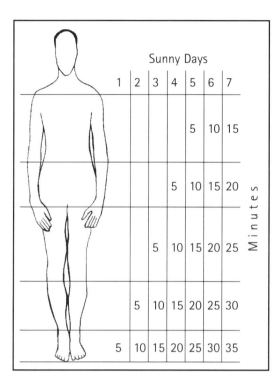

Sunny Days

1	2	3	4	5	6	7
				5	10	15
			5	10	15	20
		5	10	15	20	25
	5	10	15	20	25	30
5	10	15	20	25	30	35

Minutes

Figure 7: Diagrammatic representation of the 'Rollier Method' of sunlight therapy. The patient was covered with a white sheet. On the first day of treatment the sheet was raised to just above the ankles and the patient exposed to direct sunlight for five minutes. On the second day this exposure was repeated and the sheet raised to knee level for a further exposure of five minutes. This progression continued for about three weeks after which the full sun-bath was given. (After A. Rollier, *Heliotherapy*, London, 1923)

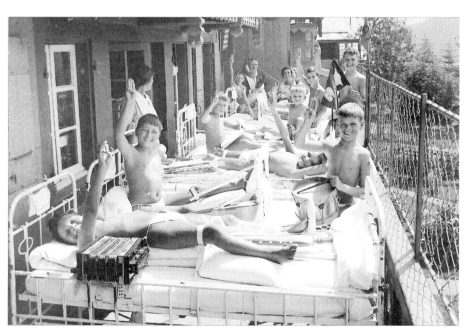

Figure 8: Patients at Dr Rollier's first heliotherapy clinic, 'Le Chalet'

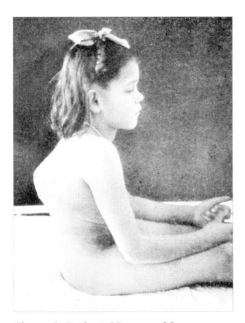

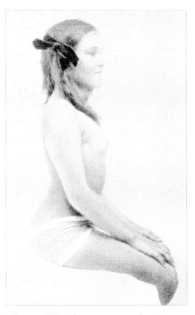

Figure 9: Patient 12 years old on arrival at Leysin. Extensive tuberculosis of the spine, paraplegia and atrophy of the muscles. Precarious general condition.

Figure 10: The same patient. Complete cure with full correction of the spine after 18 months of heliotherapy, without the use of a plaster of Paris jacket.

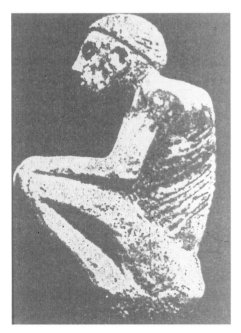

Figure 11: A small Egyptian statue of a man made of red clay which dates from around 4000 BC. The subject appears to be suffering from tuberculosis, and has the chronic pthisis, or wasting, that is a characteristic of the disease. He also has all the signs of tuberculosis of the spine which results in the large knuckle-like projection of the vertebrae and deformity of the chest which is clearly represented. It has been suggested that this statuette actually depicts an Egyptian taking a sand-bath in the sun to try and recover his health.

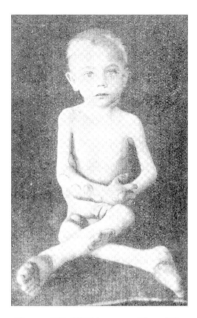 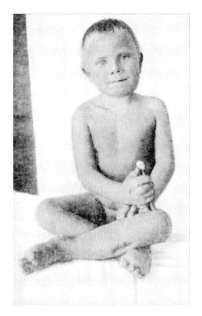

Figure 12: Child presenting 34 foci of tuberculosis on arrival at Leysin.

Figure 13: The same one year later. Full recovery, all foci of tuberculosis healed.

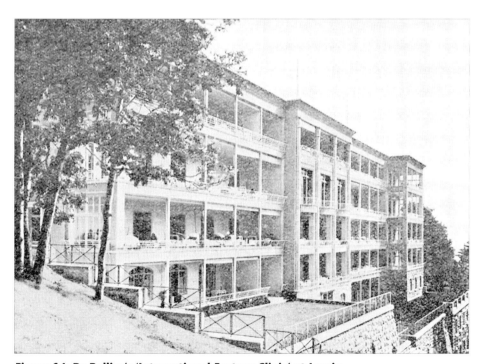

Figure 14: Dr Rollier's 'International Factory Clinic' at Leysin

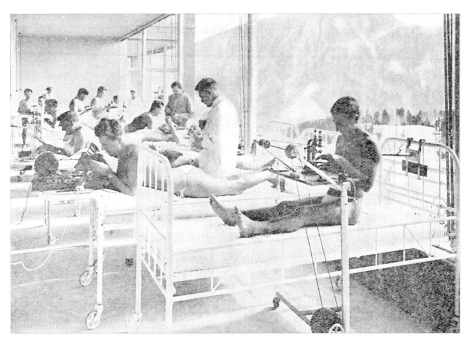

Figure 15: Patients working at the 'International Factory Clinic' while undergoing heliotherapy

THE 'ROLLIER METHOD' OF SUNBATHING FOR HEALTH

On arrival at Dr Rollier's clinic in the Alps, patients underwent a thorough medical examination. Then, after they had completed a period of acclimatization, they were carefully exposed to cold air. After one to two weeks of this open-air treatment the sunlight therapy could begin. Gradual exposure to cold air stimulated the body to produce heat and this speeded up the healing process. Cool conditions also reduced the risk of over-exposure to the sun's rays. Auguste Rollier regarded exposure to the sun at temperatures greater than 18°C, or 64°F, to be a 'hot-air bath' and not a sun-bath. As he put it in the *British Medical Journal* in 1922:

> *A very current mistake consists in thinking that the sun bath is all the more efficacious if prolonged or taken when the sun is at its hottest; this is an inconsistency against which Nature seems to warn us.*

Dr Rollier considered that the safest way to sunbathe was to begin with the feet, then the legs and arms, before exposing the abdomen and chest. By adopting this approach he could assess the tolerance of each patient to sunlight before the more sensitive parts of the body, the chest and abdomen, were uncovered. Also, if a patient received too much sunlight, only the extremities were involved. This meant that any adverse effects would be local rather than general.

His patients were wheeled out onto balconies or into solaria in their beds, wearing a loincloth and covered in a white sheet from head to toe. Their heads were covered by a hat or cloth screen. On the first day of treatment the sheet was raised to just above the ankles, and the feet exposed to the sun for just five minutes. This was repeated twice with rest-periods of ten to fifteen minutes between each sun bath. On the second day the sheet was raised to the knees, and the sun bath extended to ten minutes for each of the three sessions: the newly exposed lower legs were given five minutes and the feet ten. Exposure gradually increased so that by the fifth day of treatment the patient had three sun baths, each lasting twenty-five minutes. The feet would be uncovered first, followed by the lower legs, the thighs, the abdomen and the chest: the feet would be given the full twenty-five minutes, the legs twenty, the thighs fifteen, and so on.

For the average patient, fifteen to twenty days of the treatment were required before the entire body could be exposed from the start of the sun bath. A daily total of two to three hours of sunbathing was given in the summer months, and three to four hours in the winter. Much depended on the rate at which each patient developed a tan. After a period of about ten days their tolerance to sunlight was assessed and, if tanning was under way, the treatment had progressed well and the exposure was increased. Patients whose skin reddened rather than browned were at risk of burning, and the treatment had to proceed with great caution. Of all of the patients on whom he practised heliotherapy it was 'fair Italians', with pale skin and Titian hair, who were the most difficult to treat. They reacted so violently to the sun that he found the best approach, from the very beginning of insolation of feet and legs, was to cover the exposed parts with a layer of gauze.

Heliotherapy of this kind was developed for children and adolescents who were often very seriously ill and could not respond as well to sunlight as a healthy adult. It was for this reason that exposure was so very gradual: too much sunlight could kill them. It goes without saying that sunbathing for health in this way was very different from sunbathing simply to get a tan, and has very little in common with the way most people sunbathe today. Rollier's success with heliotherapy can be attributed to the way in which the dosage of sunlight was scrupulously graded by him according to the response and requirements of each patient. The caution with which he approached exposure of the upper body to sunlight was a particular characteristic. He believed that the sun should be dispensed 'drop by drop' when nearing the chest.

He was also insistent that a combination of hot air and sunshine was bad for any form of tuberculosis, but particularly dangerous for the pulmonary form of the disease. This is why he considered it so important to make use of the early morning sun in warm weather and why he would not allow his patients to sunbathe at midday in July and August, even if they already had a healthy tan. Dr Rollier was unusual in that he abandoned plaster of Paris casts and any other conventional forms of dressing which he considered incompatible with sunlight treatment, and developed methods of extension and fixation which permitted free access of sun and air to the body for reasons he described in his book *Heliotherapy* of 1927:

> ... a plaster of Paris dressing robs of sunlight precisely those
> parts of the body which require it most. Its results are first a
> decline and then a cessation of cutaneous function, severe
> anaemia, and not infrequently even maceration of the skin;
> further, sluggishness of nutrition in all regional tissues combined
> with a diminished excretion of metabolic end-products, the
> intensity of which processes diminishes pari passu with the
> withdrawal of sunshine.

Two aspects of Rollier's work distinguish him from other physicians who used sunlight to treat disease. Firstly he believed that sunlight was central to the treatment and could cure tuberculosis. Secondly he was strongly opposed to the use of surgery in all but the most severe cases. His revolt against the wholesale use of surgery was regarded as extreme, and his methods were not accepted for many years. Doctors had great difficulty in coming to terms with such a seemingly unscientific form of treatment. More importantly perhaps, unlike surgical intervention, slow, careful tanning of the skin offered little prospect of sudden recovery or dramatic 'cures'.

What is clear from the many articles, books and scientific papers Dr Rollier published over a forty year period, is that he and his staff at Leysin were able to transform weak, sickly tubercular patients into strong, deeply-tanned individuals who were free of the disease. He also reported success in treating a number of non-tubercular conditions including rickets, burns, varicose ulcers, osteomyelitis (an infection of the bone and bone marrow, usually by the bacterium *Staphylococcus aureus),* septic abscesses, anaemia and fractures. During the First World War he coined the expression 'le pansement solaire' — 'sun-bandage' or 'sunlight-dressing' — for the heliotherapy of wounds which he described in a book he published in 1916. Auguste Rollier practised sunlight therapy at Leysin from 1903 until well into the 1940s, and had thirty-six clinics with a total of more than a thousand beds. He had an almost religious enthusiasm for heliotherapy which led to his being described as the high-priest of a solar cult with a worldwide following.

MAKING THE MOST OF SUNLIGHT

So what can we learn from these findings? A series of short sun baths three or four times a day seems to have produced better results for tuberculosis than prolonged exposure, and the effects of sunbathing in cool conditions, when the body is trying to generate heat, are very different from when it is trying to lose it. One of the most interesting things Dr Rollier noticed during the course of his work was that sunbathing early in the morning is more beneficial than at any other time of the day. He recommended that, for the best results, in the summer months the treatment should be given between 6 am and 9 am, and at lower altitudes than the Alps even earlier still. Rollier was not alone in this: other heliotherapists of the period found the same thing, and that the best time of year to sunbathe was in the spring and early summer. Diet was another important factor. Nourishing meals were part of the treatment; and it seems reasonable to suggest that well-nourished skin responds better to sunlight than skin that is low in minerals. Certainly there is evidence to support the view that some of our current problems with sunlight, skin cancer and premature ageing stem from the deficiencies of our highly refined western diet, a subject that will be examined further in the following chapter.

SUNLIGHT AND SEA BATHING

Years ago, patients with tuberculosis of the spine or hip were often bedridden for months, if not years at a time. Normally, bedridden patients such as these experienced a gradual wasting and atrophy of the muscles because they were unable to exercise. Visitors to the heliotherapy clinics run by Dr Rollier were often surprised by the excellent muscle-tone of his bedridden tubercular patients. His work shows that a combination of sunlight and fresh air has a profound effect on the human body, even when immobilized for long periods. Rollier even called sunlight 'the best masseur'.

However, patients at his clinics who could not tan did not get better, and one observation made during the heyday of sunlight therapy, in the 1920s and 1930s, was that patients who made poor progress in the Alps sometimes did better on the coast where sunbathing was combined with sea bathing, and vice versa. The leading practitioner of heliotherapy in Britain, Sir Henry Gauvain (1878–1945), used sea bathing at a clinic on the south coast of England and, incidentally, helped to set up Canada's first solarium for TB patients on Vancouver Island in British Columbia.

Henry Gauvain was born in the Channel Island of Alderney on November 28th 1878, the eldest surviving son of Captain William Gauvain, the Receiver-General for the Island. He won a scholarship to Cambridge where he graduated with a

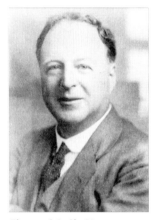

first-class degree in medicine in 1902. He went to St. Bartholomew's Hospital where he qualified in 1906, and where he served as house surgeon, midwifery assistant, and clinical assistant in the orthopaedic department before becoming Medical Superintendent of the Lord Mayor Treloar Hospital in Alton, Hampshire, which he established as a leading centre for heliotherapy.

Sir Henry Gauvain believed that sun treatment, especially in surgical tuberculosis, was particularly effective in constantly changing conditions, and that the south of England was a good location for the treatment of tuberculosis because of the varied weather and the accessibility of the sea. He found that although patients undergoing sunlight treatment inland during the early summer might rapidly improve, there came a

Figure 16: Sir Henry Gauvain (1878–1945) the leading British heliotherapist

point at which progress came to a halt. If more stimulation from sunlight was required, he had to transfer patients to the seaside where, under different conditions, with a new type of stimulus, a marked improvement was often achieved.

He found that sea bathing produced the same effect as open-air baths, but to a much greater degree. Bedridden patients who were strong enough to benefit from this rather potent treatment were first sprayed over increasing areas of the

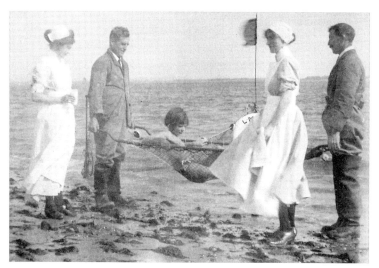

Figure 17: Sea bathing prior to sunlight therapy on the south coast of England

body with cold sea water, and then immersed in the sea for carefully graded periods of time depending on their condition. They lived so close to the sea that at high tide they could be lifted from their beds into the water. When the treatment had finished they were placed in an enclosure where they were dried and rubbed down in front of an open coke brazier. Their feet were put in hot water and they were given a hot drink, followed by a sun bath. Ambulant patients were encouraged to wade about for increasing periods of time before being sprayed with sea water and then completely immersed in the sea.

Sir Henry Gauvain noticed that each of his patients responded differently to sunlight therapy and that, even within each individual, there were both seasonal and daily variations in response. He found that his patients made the most rapid progress during the late spring and early summer. Like other heliotherapists, he also observed that morning light had the greatest therapeutic value despite being less intense than light under the midday sun. In his opinion this was because the 'light shock' of exposure to early morning sun evoked a greater response in patients than exposure later in the day. The advantages of early morning exposure were not due so much to the intensity or the nature of the light, but to the fact that exposure at this time came immediately after the darkness of night. He concluded from this observation that darkness was equally essential for sunlight treatment as light itself.

THEN AND NOW

The heliotherapy practised by Oskar Bernhard, Auguste Rollier, Sir Henry Gauvain and others enjoyed three major successes: the cure and prevention of rickets; the treatment of extrapulmonary tuberculosis; and the disinfection and healing of wounds. While sunlight played a large part in this, it was only one factor and not the whole of the regime. Exposure to pure air, freedom from fog, smoke, dust, winds and rain, combined with good nutrition, prolonged periods of rest, orthopaedic treatment and, when available, pleasant occupational therapy all played their part.

Nevertheless, the mistaken idea that sunlight, on its own, could cure tuberculosis was widely held during the 1930s. There are reports of people with the disease sunbathing without the guidance of a physician, and with no knowledge of sunlight therapy at all. It was not uncommon for someone with advanced tuberculosis of the lungs to expose the entire surface of their body, the chest included, to a combination of strong sunlight and hot humid air with disastrous consequences: haemoptesis and haemorrhage or the spread of the infection to other parts of the body. As relatively few physicians made regular use of heliotherapy, and there was little incentive for those who did not do so to become familiar with the basic principles, there was plenty of room for error. There was also a certain amount of scepticism, if not outright opposition, to the use of sunlight as a medicine. When Auguste Rollier presented the first results of his work at a conference, in Paris in 1905, it is said that the entire audience walked out. Forty years later, the distinguished British consultant surgeon and cancer specialist John Lockhart-Mummery, while writing on the relationship between medicine and magic, in his book *Nothing New Under the Sun*, felt able to dismiss sunlight therapy as follows:

> *Sunlight and ultraviolet rays are very popular just now as forms*
> *of medical treatment, but except for a very limited field they*
> *come rather under the head of pseudo-magic than scientific*
> *treatment, and most of the benefit patients get from such*
> *treatment is due to their faith in the magical results, rather*
> *than in direct benefit.*

Against this background it becomes a little clearer why the negative effects of exposure have been so widely publicized, and why the beneficial effects of sunlight on cancer and other diseases have received so little attention.

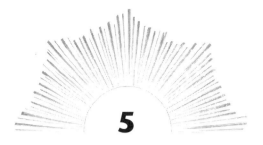

5

HOW TO SUNBATHE SAFELY

This chapter deals with the practical details of sunbathing: when, where and how to do it. A great deal remains unknown about the effects of solar radiation on the human body, but at least the findings of physicians who used it as a medicine give us a number of clues as to what to, and what not to do. They were using the sun to heal war wounds and cure tuberculosis. Their patients were in poor health and extremely sensitive to sunlight in a way that few people sunbathing today are. Nevertheless, it seems reasonable to suggest that for safe sunbathing the same basic principles apply.

The key points of heliotherapy, which are summarized below, provide a starting point for anyone wishing to sunbathe for health. In the pages that follow some of the more practical considerations are examined, such as latitude, altitude, the time of day, different times of year, ambient temperatures while sunbathing, and so on. These variables have a direct bearing on the way your body responds to sunlight and it is as well to be familiar with them. One thing they affect is your ability to generate vitamin D in the skin.

Exposing the entire body of a young white adult to a dose of ultraviolet (UV) radiation of long enough duration to cause a just perceptible reddening of the skin 24 hours after exposure (which is referred to in medical circles as a minimal erythemal dose, or 1 MED) can produce the equivalent of about 10,000 IU of vitamin D. This is far in excess of their minimum daily requirement. But it is useful nevertheless, as the human body stores vitamin D in body fat and skeletal muscle, ready to be drawn on during periods when sunlight is too weak to synthesize the vitamin.

If the minimum daily requirement is of this individual is 200 IU, then their annual requirement of vitamin D is some 73,000 IU. So, assuming they normally generate a little less vitamin D when sunbathing more moderately, say 7000 IU, then they would need 11 sessions in the sun to generate enough vitamin D for a

Table 5: Sunbathing for Health

- Plan your exposure: don't cram all of your sunbathing into two or three weeks of the year.
- If you go abroad to a hotter or colder climate; take a series of 'air-baths' for a few days before you sunbathe.
- Don't bake. The air-temperature when you sunbathe for health should be below 18°C, or 64°F.
- The most important time of year to sunbathe is in the spring and early summer.
- Early-morning sunshine seems to be particularly beneficial, so start just after dawn.
- Frequent short exposures are better than prolonged exposure to sunlight.
- It is essential to obtain the full spectrum of sunlight, so don't cover yourself with sun screen or sun block.
- Wear a hat so that the thin, sensitive skin of your face, head and neck is protected.
- If you are very sensitive to sunlight begin sunbathing the feet, then the legs, before exposing the abdomen and chest with great caution.
- If you want to tan, pay very close attention to the way your tan gradually develops. Work out your tolerance to sunlight before exposing the more sensitive parts of the body.
- Eat wholefoods, rather than refined foods
- Stay alert and, above all, do not burn.

year's supply. If only it were that simple. For one thing the current recommended daily allowance may be fine if the prevention of rickets and osteomalacia are the only aims. But for cancer prevention, or optimal bone health, double this amount of sunbathing could be required. So, in practice, arriving at a figure for the amount of sunbathing needed to meet our vitamin D requirements becomes rather complicated, if not impossible, not least because every one of us responds to sunlight in our own way.

As we have already seen, people of Asian and African origin need longer exposure times because of the increased melanin content of their skin. Someone with black skin would need the equivalent of about 6 MEDs of someone with white skin to generate the same amount of vitamin D. Of course, the more skin exposed, the more vitamin D is synthesized. Heliotherapists used to spread the exposure over the whole body, while shading the thin, sensitive skin of the head and neck. This maximizes the amount of skin exposed to the sun while protecting those areas most at risk of accelerated ageing and squamous-basal skin cancers. The face, neck and trunk are about two to four times more sensitive to the sun than the limbs, which is why they burn more easily.

Clothing prevents, or significantly impairs, the formation of vitamin D depending on the fabric worn. In tests, black wool has been shown to be very effective at blocking out the sun's rays. It stops over 98 per cent of incident UVB radiation getting through to the skin. White cotton lets about 50 per cent through, but even then several MEDs would be required before the synthesis of vitamin D could take place. In the European survey of vitamin D levels amongst 70-year-olds, referred to in chapter 3, the lowest levels were found amongst the elderly in warmer southern European countries. Wearing clothes to protect from the sun — the normal custom amongst this age group in the southern Europe — was a strong predictor of vitamin D deficiency. The condition has also been reported amongst Bedouins living in Negev desert. So clothing is a very effective barrier to UVB radiation even in the strongest sunlight.

VITAMIN D, HEALTH AND THE AGEING PROCESS

The elderly do not tolerate the heat of the sun as well as younger people. But they have a tendency to seek out warm corners in the sun if the opportunity presents itself. Indeed, older people need increasing amounts of sun exposure because the skin gradually loses its ability to produce vitamin D as it ages. The thickness of the epidermis declines with age and the amount of the vitamin D precursor 7-dehydrocholesterol declines, so by the age of 70 the skin's ability to produce vitamin D is about 30 to 50 per cent as effective as that of a twenty year old according to some estimates. So, broadly speaking, it would be advisable for older people spend time outdoors, but avoid strong sunlight because of the risk of heatstroke. Infants and young children need less vitamin D than adults and strong sunshine does not suit them. This does not mean that infants should not go out in it at all, as some experts suggest, but parents would be advised to exercise great caution when their offspring are in the sun and supervise them closely.

Another feature of the ageing process which affects vitamin D levels is that the absorption of dietary vitamin D via the intestines becomes less efficient in older people. However, vitamin D activated by sunlight bypasses any gastro-intestinal vitamin D malabsorption, and any risk of toxicity. So for these, and reasons already discussed, exposure to the sun is a better option than oral supplements for many elderly people.

The way we respond to sunshine also depends very much on our state of health. People who are well can tolerate sunshine far better than the sick or infirm. Some sick people can benefit greatly from careful exposure to sunlight, while others suffer from conditions for which sunlight is contraindicated. Very ill people sometimes have to be kept in total darkness because they are so sensitive to light. Anyone on immunosuppressive drugs should be very careful in sunlight because of their increased susceptibility to skin cancer. Also, some drugs such as carbamazepine, phenytoin, and rifampin, impair the activation of vitamin D or accelerate its clearance from the body, while chronic liver and kidney diseases can cause vitamin D deficiency. Another point to bear in mind is that healthy, well-nourished skin seems to respond better to sunlight than skin that lacks nutrients or which contains abnormally high levels of fat, a subject examined at the end of this chapter.

TIME OF DAY AND TIME OF YEAR

One of the most significant things that the physicians who used sunlight as a medicine remarked on during the course of their work was that sunbathing early in the morning is more beneficial than at any other time of the day. They recommended that sunlight treatment should be given in the first few hours for the best results, unless they were disinfecting wounds where stronger sunlight was needed, or treating rheumatism or other conditions where the body needed to be warmed. In countries at northerly latitudes such as Britain, UVB radiation with the right wavelengths to produce vitamin D in the skin is only present at ground level from about 9 a.m. to 3 p.m., in the six months from April to September. Early morning sunlight may not be strong enough to synthesize vitamin D in the skin, but this seems to be the best time of day to begin exposure of skin which is not used to sunlight. Certainly sufferers of SAD seem to benefit from light at this time of day, and there may be some as yet unexplained connection between these psychological and physiological phenomena.

Dr Auguste Rollier, Dr Oskar Bernhard, and Sir Henry Gauvain all found that the best time of year to sunbathe for health was in the spring and early summer. Sunbathing in the spring prepares the body for stronger sunlight during the summer months, and in the spring and summer that vitamin D is synthesized in the skin. But there may be other, as yet unexplained, forces at work which require us to make the most of periods of growth and expansion — spring and early

114

summer — to utilize health-giving sunlight to its fullest extent. Our ancestors had to attune themselves to its natural cycles in order to survive, and our physiological and psychological requirements are much the same as theirs. So it is to our advantage to become familiar with the sun's path through the heavens, and the solar year, if for no other reason than the amount of solar radiation available for sunbathing varies depending on the time of day and the seasons.

THE SOLAR CALENDAR

Three types of calendar have been used down the centuries; the lunar, solar and lunisolar. The lunar calendar is based on the phases of the moon. The solar calendar is based on the apparent motion of the sun through the heavens and the lunisolar calendar is a combination of the two. The oldest and at one time the most widely used is the lunar calendar which has 13 lunar months of about 29.5 days' duration. It is relatively straightforward to work out where you are in a lunar month simply by watching the moon wax and wane. However, the lunar year is roughly 19 days longer than the solar year of just over 365 days. More sophisticated calendars combined the lunar month and solar year, even though there is no exact relationship between the two. The correct term for the discrepancy in days between the solar and lunar years is the 'epact'.

THE SOLAR YEAR

For those of us who live in the northern hemisphere the shortest day, or the winter solstice, falls on the 21st of December. The longest day, or summer solstice, falls on the 21st of June — half a year later. The position of sunrise and sunset on these two days set the limits of the sun's apparent motion throughout the year: the sun rises and sets at its northernmost limit on midsummer's day and its southernmost limit at midwinter.

On the morning of the winter solstice in the south of England the sun rises in the southeast a few minutes after 8 a.m. By noon it has reached an angle of 15 degrees above the horizon and it sets in the southwest just before 4 p.m. On the morning of the summer solstice the sun rises in the northeast at 3.43 a.m. By noon it has reached an angle of 62 degrees above the horizon and it sets in the northwest just after 8.20 p.m.

So if you can find somewhere that faces south which you can visit at noon throughout the year you will notice that on June the 21st the sun will be almost overhead, and there will be about sixteen hours of daylight. The sun will have come around from behind your left shoulder and will disappear behind your right shoulder as the day draws in. On December the 21st there will only be eight hours of daylight and the sun will be closer to the southern horizon at noon than at any other time of the year.

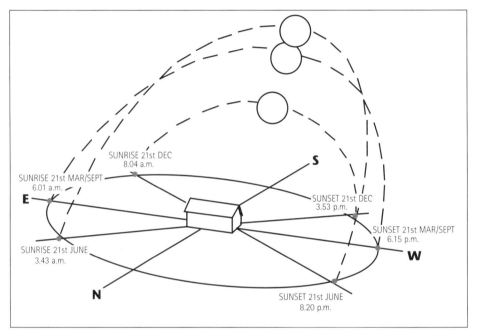

Figure 18: Sunpath diagram for latitude 51.5 degrees

The equinoxes are the two occasions in the year when day and night are of equal length. Sunrise is due east and sunset due west, and the sun reaches an angle of about 40 degrees to the horizon. The vernal equinox on about the 21st of March marks the onset of spring, while the autumn equinox takes place on the 22nd or 23rd of September. One thing that is noticeable about the equinoxes is that the length of each day changes much more quickly at this time of year than it does around midsummer and midwinter. For example, at the latitude of London (about 51.5 degrees) on the 7th of December the length of day is only four minutes longer than on midwinter's day on December the 21st. Similarly, two weeks before and after June the 21st each day is only about eight minutes shorter than is June the 21st itself. But on March the 7th, two weeks before the spring equinox, the day is forty-five minutes shorter than it is on March the 21st. Two weeks later, on April the 4th, it is nearly an hour longer.

116

Another thing to bear in mind is that the seasons of the year do not coincide with the major points of the solar calendar. Midsummer's day is not in the middle of summer, nor is midwinter's day in the middle of winter. In fact, the four seasons of what used to be known as the 'farmer's year' — spring, summer, autumn and winter — are a month later than they should be. To illustrate the point, if we take each of the three-month periods that make a season and space them equally about the four principal positions of the sun — midsummer, midwinter and the equinoxes — then summer would correspond to the months of May, June and July. But the farmer's summer is June, July and August, even though the sun is at its highest point in the sky in June. So, although the apparent paths of the sun across the heavens in May and July, or in April and August, may be identical, their effects on the human body could be very different, as the historical evidence seems to suggest.

LATITUDE AND ALTITUDE

The strength of UVB radiation at ground level is determined by the elevation of the sun relative to the horizon. This angle governs the length of the path that the sun's ultraviolet ray's have to travel through the ozone layer, and then through the earth's atmosphere, before they reach us. The longer the path, the greater the absorption and scattering of UVB radiation. More UVB radiation is present at midday than either the early morning or late afternoon, because at midday the sun is high in the sky and the path of its rays through the atmosphere is shortened. Similarly, the nearer you are to the equator, and the higher you are above sea level, the stronger solar radiation becomes. Solar radiation only has to pass through about half as much of the atmosphere to reach the equator as it does to reach polar regions. On the ground, UVB radiation is approximately four times as strong at the equator as it is at the Arctic and Antarctic circles, and as far as altitude is concerned, radiation increases by about 10 per cent for each mile above sea level.

The amount of ultraviolet radiation that reaches the earth's surface also depends on the amount of dust, haze and water vapour in the atmosphere. This complicates matters because variations in cloud cover and atmospheric pollution influence the transmission of UVB radiation far more than they do the transmission of visible light. This means that it is very difficult to judge how much UVB radiation is present in sunlight on the basis of how bright it is at ground level, and the only way to really find out how strong ultraviolet radiation levels are is to make direct measurements with a UVB monitor, or pay very close attention to the way your skin responds to it. A very crude measure of the strength of the sun is to look at the length of shadows during the course of each day. Roughly speaking, if the shadow you cast is shorter than your height, then you are in strong sunlight.

Clouds present a particular problem to the sunbather because the water in clouds filters out solar infrared radiation much more effectively than it does ultraviolet radiation. So the 'heat' of the sun is diminished while most of the UVB gets through. In practical terms this means that under clouds one gets a sensation of heat normally associated with weak rather than strong sunlight, and it is easy to assume that UVB levels are correspondingly low when they may not be. Speaking from personal experience, it takes very little time to burn under light cloud during the middle of the day in the Canary Islands — providing you have the right skin type and are not tanned already. Under heavy clouds the ultraviolet component of sunlight is reduced by 30 per cent or more, and storm clouds can block out most of it.

AIR POLLUTION

Air pollution can be a very effective barrier to UVB radiation. In the 18th and 19th century, the widespread combustion of coal with a high sulphur content resulted in low levels of ultraviolet radiation for many town and city dwellers. The smoke and sulphurous gases produced when coal was burned filtered it out. Today, in developed countries at least, the problem of air pollution is usually associated with the exhaust fumes from motor cars, although in Britain about half the nation's energy use provides heating and other services for buildings. So the gas, oil, and coal-fired boilers in buildings, both big and small, contributes to pollution in urban areas.

Urban air pollution is a highly complex mixture of vapours, particles and gases some of which, such as hydrocarbons, oxides of nitrogen and atmospheric oxygen, react with sunlight to form what is known as photochemical smog. A major constituent of photochemical smog is ozone which is, as we have seen already, an effective filter of ultraviolet radiation. In a city surrounded by hills or mountains, air pollution can be very severe and is it is made worse by sunlight. Anyone who is used to sunbathing in urban areas should be aware that if they move to a rural, alpine or seaside location they will get more ultraviolet radiation simply because the air is cleaner.

SURROUNDINGS

The surrounding environment has a major influence on the intensity of ultraviolet radiation incident on the skin. Fresh snow reflects up to 85 per cent of the UVB radiation that hits it, and old snow some 50 per cent. Dry white sand reflects some 17 per cent and wet sand 9 percent. Grass reflects only 2–3 per cent. Building materials and rendered surfaces reflect significant amounts of UV, up to as much as 50 per cent. Even on a patio in the shade of an umbrella there is scope for tanning and burning if the sunlight is strong enough. Water reflects only 5 per cent of the UVB radiation that strikes it, but is very transparent to it, therefore shallow water offers very little protection from the sun's rays.

AMBIENT TEMPERATURE

One sensible precaution which anyone can take when they start sunbathing is to do so at air temperatures of around 18°C or 64°F. From what is known of the work of Auguste Rollier and other heliotherapists, it was sunbathing in cool conditions which speeded up the metabolism rather than depressing it, and this had a beneficial effect on tuberculosis patients. It seems to have strengthened their immune systems and stimulated the self-healing powers of the body. The reasons for this are not altogether clear, but it would certainly seem to be the safest approach to sunbathing unless you are very sensitive to cold conditions.

When air temperatures are high there is almost certainly a correspondingly high level of ultraviolet radiation. So, as a broad rule-of-thumb, exposure at around 25°C or about 80°F should be avoided by anyone whose skin is not used to very strong sunlight. Also, never sunbathe in a breeze because the cooling effect on the body can give the impression that the intensity of the sun is less than it actually is. Always sunbathe in a sheltered spot where air movement over the body is negligible. Even if the temperature is low, or the wind makes you feel cold, the sun's ultraviolet radiation can still be very strong.

DIET AND THE SUN

In Chapter 2 reference was made to the influence vitamins and minerals in the diet have on the way human skin responds to sunlight. One component of the western diet which may also affect skin exposed to the sun's rays is fat. The American nutritionist and sunlight therapist Dr Zane Kime was in no doubt about this:

Unless one has a proper diet, sunlight has an ill effect on the skin. This must be emphasized: sunbathing is dangerous for those who are on the standard high-fat American diet or do not get an abundance of vegetables, whole grains and fresh fruits. Those on the standard high-fat diet should stay out of the sun and protect themselves from it; but at the same time they will suffer the consequences of both the high-fat diet and the deficiency of sunlight.

Dr Zane Kime, 'Sunlight Could Save Your Life'

Dr Kime wrote this in 1980 and, in the intervening period, his views on the dangers of combining excessive fat consumption and sunbathing have, to some extent, been confirmed. But before we examine the relationship between sunlight exposure and fat in the diet, there are broader health issues to address concerning the fat in our food. A diet high in fat is considered to increase the likelihood of obesity, hypertension, diabetes and gallbladder disease. Studies also suggest that there may be an association between a high dietary fat intake and major internal cancers such as colon, breast, prostate and ovarian cancer. But it is still not known whether lowering fat intake to levels found in countries that have lower incidences of these cancers reduces the risks of developing them, nor is it by any means certain that a low-fat diet, on its own, will reduce the prevalence of obesity and the chronic diseases which accompany it. The same applies to coronary heart disease. Death rates from coronary heart disease are much lower in southern European countries than in north-western Europe; but a Mediterranean diet appears to offer little protection to people living in northern European who adopt it, unless they already have heart disease and wish to lower their cholesterol levels.

In newly industrialized countries, such as China, and in Central America cancers, cardiovascular disease and diabetes are emerging on a scale that was unexpected only a few years ago. In South-East Asia breast and colo-rectal cancer, which were almost unknown twenty or thirty years ago, are becoming significant problems. Breast cancer has become a cause for concern in the Middle East, Egypt and Iran. Western lifestyles, which include high-fat diets and low levels of physical activity, seem to bring these 'diseases of affluence' with them. The foods which it is said could prevent as much as 40 per cent of all cancers — whole grains, vegetables, fruits, pastas and pulses rather than meat and fat — are the staple ingredients of diets in the developing world, and it is this type of diet that multinational fast-food chains and western food companies are so effective at undermining.

One factor in the emergence of the 'diseases of affluence' in developing countries could be lack of sunlight. If the change to a western diet is accompanied by lifestyle changes that include the adoption of western-style work patterns, with more time spent indoors, there could be fewer opportunities to get out in the sun. As discussed in Chapter 3, heart disease may be brought on by sunlight deficiency, only to be made worse by high levels of cholesterol in the blood. A similar process could underlie the development of breast and colon cancer, when an immune system weakened by lack of sunlight, fresh air and exercise is subjected to a diet high in fat and low in fibre, fruit and vegetables. Then again, the type of fat being eaten in developing countries as they adopt western dietary habits may be causing health problems.

Is Fat a Sunbathing Issue?

Our ancestors ate a combination of saturated animal fat, the polyunsaturated fats which occur naturally in fish and vegetables, and olive oil when and where it was available. They did not eat oil that had been refined, or processed industrially, as many of us do today. It is only in the last hundred years or so that polyunsaturated fats have been extracted from corn, seeds and beans in the form of refined oils, either mechanically or with chemical solvents. In recent years these refined fats have been promoted as healthy alternatives to saturated fats because they reduce cholesterol levels.

As these refined oils are liquid at room temperature they cannot be used as a spread for sandwiches or shortening for baking. To get around this problem an industrial process called partial hydrogenation was developed to make polyunsaturated fats solid or semi-solid at normal temperatures. In this process hydrogen gas is added to the unsaturated part of the oil in the presence of a catalyst, at temperatures of around $200^{\circ}C$.

Polyunsaturated fats are radically altered during the hydrogenation process, becoming trans fats. Although hydrogenation makes these fat molecules appear similar to the fatty acids in olive oil, which is the healthiest oil for cooking, industrially produced trans-fatty acids do not share the same healthy properties. Nevertheless, the production of partially hydrogenated fats has risen steadily during the course of this century because of their low cost and suitability for deep frying. They also oxidize more slowly than liquid oils, which means they have a longer shelf life.

For many years there has been concern that trans fats may cause increased atherosclerosis and other diseases such as cancer. In 1985 a comprehensive report was issued which did not find any clear evidence of adverse effects, but more recent epidemiological studies have shown that the intake of partially hydrogenated fats is associated with an increased risk of coronary heart disease. Researchers have found that trans-fatty acids in some margarines and fried snacks cause an increase of a type of cholesterol which leads to the clogging of arteries. The increase in this harmful cholesterol, called low-density lipoprotein (LDL), is accompanied by a decrease of another type of cholesterol called high-density lipoprotein (HDL), which seem to protect against arterial disease. HDL absorbs excess LDL molecules and takes them back to the liver where they are turned into waste. Saturated fats increase both LDL and HDL, which means that saturated animal fats are actually less harmful than the trans-fatty acids in products which are supposed to offer a healthier alternative to them.

It has also emerged that there may be a link between trans-fatty acids and breast cancer. Although research in this area is in its very early stages, the results of a Europe-wide study on nutrition and breast cancer discussed in the *American Journal of Clinical Nutrition* in 1997, found that women most at risk from the disease had higher than normal amounts of trans-fatty acids in their body fat. It is not easy to establish a direct association between cancer and a specific ingredient in the diet, but if trans fats do increase the risk of breast cancer, or heart disease, then there are good grounds for using only unhydrogenated vegetable oils for baking and frying, and avoiding commercial products which are baked or fried in hydrogenated fats. This means cutting out crisps, chips, doughnuts, biscuits and the like. It also means reducing the intake of products that are sold on the basis that they are 'low in saturated fats' or 'low in cholesterol' but which contain trans fats. This is not always easy, as food labelling is not always as informative as it could be.

DIET AND SKIN CANCER

As long ago as 1939 it was shown that cancer tumours induced by ultraviolet radiation developed more rapidly in animals fed high levels of dietary fat than in animals receiving lower levels of fat. In 1995 an article published in the *International Journal of Cancer* showed that a low-fat diet could be a major factor in the prevention and management of non-melanoma skin cancers in humans. During a two-year study, a group of skin cancer patients were put on a low-fat diet to see if this had any influence on their condition. They were instructed to limit the amount of fat they ate to 20 per cent of their total calorific intake, while other patients taking part in the experiment were left to eat, on average, 38 per cent of their calorific intake as fat. At the end of the experiment patients in the low-fat group had significantly fewer cancers than patients who had made no changes to their diet. Research has also shown that a low-fat diet can reduce the incidence of actinic keratoses, the premalignant skin lesions which can develop into squamous cell carcinoma. If, as it appears, a reduction in the amount of calories consumed in the form of fat of whatever type from 40 per cent to 20 per cent can affect the occurrence of basal cell and squamous cell carcinoma, Dr Kime's warnings about sunlight exposure for those on a high-fat, low-nutrient diet appear justified. Given the scale of the problem — in 1995 some 1.2 million cases of basal cell carcinoma were diagnosed and treated in the USA alone — more needs to be done to alert people to the dangers of combining a high-fat diet and sunlight exposure.

As yet, the relationship between skin cancer and the consumption of trans fats or refined polyunsaturated fats has not been investigated to any great extent. Certainly the type of fat one eats subsequently appears in the tissues, including the skin, and as the proportion of fat increases in the diet, it also increase in the tissues. Whether trans fats or, for that matter, refined polyunsaturated fats play a part in the genesis of skin cancer remains open to question. But it now seems clear that adopting a low-fat diet can reduce the occurrence of non-melanoma skin cancers.

In fact, diet therapy has long been an alternative, if little known, option for cancer sufferers. There is one particularly striking account of this approach being used to cure the most dangerous form of skin cancer, malignant melanoma. Beata Bishop, in her book *A Time to Heal*, describes how she recovered from malignant melanoma by following a strict dietary regime. A mole on her leg had become malignant and she underwent surgery. Although the focus of the disease was removed and she was assured that her problems were over, within a year the cancer had spread to her lymphatic system. She faced the prospect of further extensive surgery with an uncertain outcome, or death within a few months if she did nothing. Ms Bishop chose an alternative therapy in which optimal nutrition and detoxification were used to restore her damaged immune system to the point where it could destroy the malignancy. The regime she followed was originally developed by the distinguished German physician Dr Max Gerson, and is described in his book *A Cancer Therapy — Results of Fifty Cases*. Dr Gerson's diet includes the fresh juices of organically grown fruits, leaves and vegetables; vegetarian food; and frequent detoxification. It excludes many of the ingredients normally found in a typical western diet, particularly salt.

Followers of Dr Gerson's regime are encouraged to get out in the sun early in the morning, or in the evening. They are to remove their glasses if they wear them, and stimulate their pineal glands with the full spectrum of the sun's rays.

However, sunbathing plays no part in the therapy and, significantly, it appears to have played no part in the genesis of Beata Bishop's melanoma either. Indeed, it is tempting to speculate that lack of sunlight may have been a contributory factor. In her book she recounts that the eminent dermatologist who first diagnosed her melanoma suggested that sunlight might be the cause, and how she disagreed with this hypothesis as she disliked sunbathing.

Beata Bishop's secondary cancer was diagnosed in 1980, yet she is alive and well despite what was a very gloomy prognosis at the time. This remarkable recovery flies in the face of much conventional thinking on melanoma, diet, cancer and much else besides. The therapy which she used with such success is one of a number of alternatives to chemotherapy and surgery, and many of these unorthodox treatments are reviewed in Jonathan Chamberlain's book *Fighting Cancer*. None of these alternative approaches uses sunlight to any extent, and so Drs Zane Kime, John Ott and Auguste Rollier appear to be the only therapists to publish evidence in its favour.

As we saw in Chapter 3, when Dr Kime was treating a patient with breast cancer he encouraged her to eliminate refined polyunsaturated fat from her diet. Polyunsaturated fats are essential to the body because they produce molecules called prostaglandins which regulate nerve signalling and muscle movement. But in their refined form they, like saturated and unsaturated fats, encourage the formation of free radicals. A number of vitamins, minerals and compounds are known to be capable of either preventing free radicals from forming, or protecting the body from damage once free radicals have formed. They are found in whole foods, but are not as abundant in foods once they have been refined. Polyunsaturated fat in its refined form is stripped of many of these ingredients, so it is possible that the consumption of refined polyunsaturated fats, which have been promoted as a healthy alternative to saturated fats, has contributed to the increase in skin cancers seen in the last few decades. Be that as it may, a low-fat diet does seem to inhibit the recurrence of basal cell carcinoma, while an increase in vitamin intake may have similar benefits.

SUNBATHING FOR HEALTH: WHICH DIET?

Having looked briefly at the impact of diet on cancer and the skin, we now come to the rather daunting task of identifying exactly what constitutes a healthy diet for sunbathing. There are those who argue that, physiologically, human beings still belong in the Stone Age. As such, we should eat the diet of our hunter-gatherer ancestors if we really want to stay healthy. This means a diet of wild game, fresh fish, and uncultivated fruit and vegetables, such as berries, tubers and nuts. Hunter-gatherers eat little or no cereals and no dairy foods, while sugar, salt and fat are hard for them to come by. The urban diet contains these ingredients in abundance, yet we still behave like our ancestors — as if fat, salt and sugar are in short supply — which may explain why the western diet poses such a threat to world health.

The hand-to-mouth Stone Age diet is, if you like, a starting point. The Chinese diet represents the opposite end of the nutritional spectrum in terms of its variety and sophistication. Diet therapy has long formed part of folk medicine in China, and the Chinese have gone to great lengths to define the medical properties of foods so that they can use them to prevent disease and treat chronic ailments cheaply and effectively. Their civilization has the greatest range of food products and ways of preparing them known to history. They believe that a wide variety of foods is necessary to maintain health, and that a diet which is balanced, in their terms, will restore or maintain a state of harmony. To the Chinese, health is something rather more profound than the absence of disease. It is a state of internal harmony which puts the individual in tune with the constant changes that take place in the immediate environment, and beyond. They classify foods according to their 'heating' or 'cooling' properties, a practice which formed part of ancient Greek medicine.

The classification of 'hot' or 'cold' does not refer to the temperature of the foodstuff itself but to its ability to heat up or cool down the body. Hot foods are so called because if taken in excess they cause 'hot' symptoms such as fevers, sweating, flushing, dry throat, dry lips and inflammation. Cold foods help to cure hot diseases by reducing body temperature, but an inappropriate diet of cooling foods would produce, amongst other symptoms, chills, stomach upsets, wasting and general lassitude. Chinese dietary theory advocates a balance of heating and cooling foods, but stresses that the composition varies from person to person according to their constitution and whatever ails them. Each person has a different degree of heat or cold in their make-up, and this will vary during different stages of life or illness. Broadly speaking, a hot person would tend to be energetic and firmly built with a florid complexion, and would not feel the cold. In contrast, a cold person is sensitive to the cold, may be weak or emaciated in appearance, and is lacking in energy with a tendency to develop cold disorders. The classification of foods, and even people, into categories of hot and cold is synonymous with the ancient Chinese duality of yin and yang, which is the foundation of Chinese medicine.

In practice, Chinese diet therapy conforms to the same principles which underlie Chinese herbal medicine, and it is entirely compatible with the other therapies that constitute the traditional Chinese medical canon, such as acupuncture and remedial exercise. If you fall ill and consult a practitioner, he or she may well prescribe a course of herbs or acupuncture, and advise you to change your diet. You may also be told to repeat a specific exercise many times each day if you wish to be restored to health. So the Chinese diet is unusual in that it forms part of a fully integrated medical system, which includes exercise. This is the complete opposite of the western model in which nutrition comes much lower on the list of priorities.

The Chinese view of healthy eating is very much at odds with some of the modern thinking on diet in the West, which recommends that fruit and vegetables should be eaten raw so that all of the vitamins and minerals contained in them can be fully absorbed. Although a limited amount of raw food can be beneficial, the Chinese consider that a disproportionate amount of this 'cold-energy' food will weaken the spleen and will be difficult to digest, so they are cautious about consuming salads, fruit, iced drinks and ice cream in large quantities. Also, to the Chinese, a healthy lifestyle is one in which diet and exercise are tailored to the needs of the individual, taking into account personal and family health histories. This is very much the opposite of the one-size-fits-all mentality that underlies much of the current thinking on nutrition and exercise in developed countries. There is now a bewildering choice of diets on offer in the West for anyone interested in improving their nutritional status. If this were not confusing enough, there is also the vexed question of whether the routine use of dietary supplements is good or bad. Some experts say yes, while others insist that a diet tailored to suit individual needs based on wholefoods will supply the necessary vitamins perfectly well. But if you come from a family with a history of osteoporosis, or are in any way at risk of developing the disease, there is a good case for adding mineral supplements to your diet and taking cod-liver oil during the winter months if you can't get some ultraviolet radiation.

Clearly, anyone who wishes to sunbathe for health needs to take a careful look at what they eat, and a consultation with a nutritionist may be in order if there is a tendency for some of the 'diseases of affluence' to occur in your family. One thing that should be restated is that a wholefood diet was an integral part of Dr Rollier's heliotherapy. His patients were fed on a mixture of fresh vegetables and grains with some dairy produce, very little meat and no alcohol. Dr Zane Kime, in his book on sunlight and health recommended much the same thing, and at the present time a low-fat, high-fibre diet with plenty of fruit, vegetables, whole grains, lean meat, fish and low-fat dairy products is widely advocated. The British government now advises us to eat five portions of fruit and vegetables a day which, on the face of it, seems a very sensible recommendation. However, there are those who would argue that the range and amount of pesticides now used during the production of conventionally grown produce means that this may not be as healthy an option as it seems.

Despite reassurances to the effect that the levels of pesticide residues in fruit and vegetables are not a cause for concern, little is known about the combined effects of eating foods which contain different pesticides in varying amounts. Unfortunately, recent history suggests that the needs of consumers assume rather less importance in the great scheme of things than the interests of producers. So whichever diet you decide to pursue, there is a very good case for including organic produce whenever you can. Your body will have fewer chemicals to deal with, and you may reduce your chances of being exposed to drug-resistant bacteria.

SUNLAMPS AND SOLARIA

In the clinics where heliotherapy was practised there was often a ward or a room set aside for 'artificial' sunlight. During periods of bad weather patients could continue their treatment with the aid of ultraviolet radiation from lamps. The first of these was designed by Niels Finsen and they became very popular amongst the medical profession in the years before the introduction of antibiotics. To heliotherapists such machines were useful, but very much a second best to sunlight, as these lamps did not reproduce accurately the natural spectrum of the sun's rays.

The modern sunbed has received a considerable amount of adverse publicity, and much of it is justified. Certainly, the pursuit of the 'fast tan' and the 'year-round tan' may have done users more harm than good, as tanning for cosmetic purposes is very different from sunbathing for health. If one is going to use an artificial source of radiation to get a tan, then it should be as close as possible to the natural spectrum of the sun's rays. In recent years sunbeds have been marketed on the basis that they differ from natural sunlight in that they emit a high proportion of UVA radiation. This was thought to be safer than UVB, but is now known to be highly penetrative and responsible for photoageing. Prolonged exposure to any form of radiation can be hazardous but it is more likely to be so if it differs markedly from something as natural as sunlight.

Niels Finsen, who pioneered the artificial light bath, always used to insist on low air temperatures for his tuberculosis patients. Like the heliotherapists who followed in his footsteps, Finsen found that this produced the best results. As we have already seen, air temperature may well be a factor in the development of skin cancer. So lying down in a warm solarium and getting a rapid tan from a sunbed which emits predominantly UVA, has little to recommend it. Where sun-tanning equipment is useful is as a reliable source of ultraviolet radiation for those of us who want to keep a moderate level of exposure and are unable to get out in the sun. Exposure to ultraviolet radiation, especially in winter months, can prevent vitamin D deficiency and disease. The amount required depends on a number of factors, most of which have already been discussed, and it is not necessary to tan to get the benefits.

Ten minutes in front of a full-spectrum sunlamp two or three times a week may be all that is needed to increase immunity to infectious and degenerative diseases. By the same token, exposure to winter sunlight may have a beneficial influence on general health. In Britain, sunlight at this time of year may not be strong enough to produce vitamin D in the skin, but the therapeutic effects of exposure to the natural spectrum of the sun's rays probably extend well beyond vitamin D synthesis. Certainly, as we saw in a previous chapter, winter sunlight should bring some relief from the symptoms of seasonal affective disorder, and it seems to prevent multiple sclerosis.

In order to sunbathe in the autumn and winter months one has to be in a sheltered spot, out of the wind. Indeed, one of the golden rules of sunbathing is to make sure that air movement over the body is minimized. Probably the best way to do this, during the winter months at least, is to construct some form of revolving solarium. In the pre-war years it was not unknown for a light-therapy patient to be issued with a shed for their garden or allotment which could follow the 'round of the sun'. Two famous literary figures had something along these lines. George Bernard Shaw did his writing in a small garden shed which was on a turntable. The Roman author, Pliny the Younger (62–113 AD), had a winter residence that had a solarium. This was a permanent structure which could not be moved around but was part of a villa which was designed to capture the rays of the winter sun.

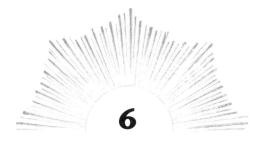

6

INDOORS, OUTDOORS

As with so many other areas of human activity, medicine and architecture are subject to the vagaries of fashion. Routine procedures and long-cherished beliefs can soon become outmoded or obsolete in the light of new thinking. Unfortunately, when a new paradigm or philosophy appears it is sometimes accompanied by a desire to break with the past altogether. This happened in architecture at the beginning of the 20th century when the pioneers of the Modern Movement attempted to sweep away all that had gone before. New methods of construction and new materials allowed them to make a radical departure from previous styles of building. The constraints imposed by masonry construction no longer applied as, for the first time, steel and pre-stressed concrete beams enabled them to span wide spaces. This meant that windows could become continuous openings in the building envelope. Balconies could be constructed with little difficulty and pitched roofs could be dispensed with. Thanks to these and other developments, which we will look at in a moment, a new aesthetic emerged to become what we now know as modern architecture. Western medicine underwent something along similar lines in the 1950s when antibiotics became available. Suddenly doctors had drugs at their disposal which could cure, in hours or days, infections that would have taken months of hospital care to overcome. Medical practice underwent changes as radical in their own way as those in architecture.

Dislocations of this kind have many consequences, for good and ill, and one of them is that the past often has to be learnt again, the wheel reinvented. It is with this in mind that the following pages have been written, in an attempt to highlight a few forgotten truths about sunlight, health and the indoor environment.

The idea that buildings that admit sunlight are in some way healthier than those that exclude it is a very ancient one. As the old Italian proverb points out

'Dove non va il sole, va il medico' or *'Where the sun does not go, the doctor does'.* This saying may well have been coined during the early days of Imperial Rome, when solar architecture, sun-worship and sunlight therapy went hand in hand. To the Romans, solar architecture would have been entirely compatible with their ideas about medicine and their religious beliefs, as anyone familiar with the writings of Vitruvius will know.

During the reign of Augustus in the first century BC, Marcus Vitruvius Pollio, the Roman military engineer and architect, wrote his famous *Ten Books on Architecture.* Although later European architecture owes a great deal to the principles set out by Vitruvius in this highly influential text, his recommendations on the education of architects, on their responsibilities towards the health of the occupants of their buildings and on solar design were not embraced as enthusiastically as other aspects of his work; for example, the classic principles of harmony, proportion and symmetry.

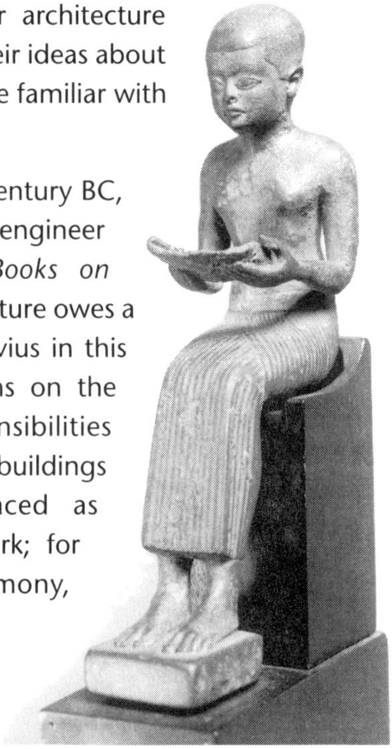

Vitruvius felt that the true architect should be able to demonstrate a working knowledge of a number of subjects including mathematics, geometry, optics, acoustics, astronomy, philosophy, history, law and, significantly, medicine. Knowledge of medicine was essential if an architect was to be able to select healthy sites both for cities and for the buildings within the city walls. Vitruvius believed that careful design of public buildings such as theatres and temples

Figure 19: Imhotep (fl 2980–2950 BC), who personifies the association between medicine, architecture and sun-worship. Imhotep is the first physician known to history, and one of the world's great architects. He supervised the construction of the Egyptian's first pyramid together with a temple to their sun-god Horus.

prevented illness, and that street planning could actually help cure chronic sicknesses such as tuberculosis.

According to Vitruvius, architects had to know how to choose a healthy site for a temple so as to favour the gods of healing. Having done so, they then had to ensure that the temple had the correct orientation so that supplicants would face the rising sun during their devotions. On a more mundane level, Vitruvius describes how the solar architecture of dwellings should be adapted to suit the different climates of the Roman Empire:

> *One type of house seems appropriate to build in Egypt, another in Spain… one still different in Rome, and so on with lands and countries of other characteristics. This is because one part of the earth is directly under the sun's course, another is far away from it, while another lies midway between these two… it is obvious that designs for houses ought similarly to conform to the nature of the country and to diversities of climate.*
>
> *Vitruvius 'On Architecture'*

Obvious, maybe, but with the fall of Rome, and the end of sunlight therapy, the principles of solar design were largely ignored or forgotten. Doctors no longer thought that sunlight was important to health, and so there was no reason for architects to believe so either. Consequently, the advantages of getting solar radiation into buildings to prevent disease and, for that matter, save energy were not appreciated in much of urban Europe for more than a thousand years. So-called 'folk' architecture continued to demonstrate the principles described by Vitruvius, but city dwellers were largely deprived of the sun. Matters were made worse in England by the Window Tax and compounded by a tax on glass. The Window Tax was imposed in 1695 with the result that windows were bricked up and houses were often designed with the minimum of fenestration to avoid payment. The tradition of inadequate windows extended well beyond the abolition of this tax in 1851.

While legislators may have been ignorant of the relationship between sunlight, ventilation and occupant wellbeing during this period, high levels of natural light were encouraged in hospitals by a few enlightened individuals, including Florence Nightingale (1820–1910). Miss Nightingale is best remembered as 'The Lady of the Lamp' because of the way she cared for the sick and wounded at the infamous military hospitals at Scutari, during the Crimean War. What is not so well known about her is that she went on to become an international authority on the design of hospitals. Florence Nightingale was unusual amongst designers in that she considered sunlight and fresh air to be of the utmost importance in providing a healthy environment for the sick, and she was responsible for some of the first sunlit hospital wards.

Fortunately, as the therapeutic and sanitary properties of the sun's rays began to be investigated on a scientific basis, sunlight came to be more widely appreciated. In 1877, Arthur Downes and Thomas Blunt made their discovery that sunlight has a bactericidal property, and then in 1890 Robert Koch showed that sunlight was lethal to the bacterium which caused the disease. These discoveries had profound implications for architects and designers.

BUILDINGS AND BACTERIA

Once it was finally recognized that tuberculosis bacteria were present in the mucus or phlegm of infected individuals, and that dried tuberculous sputum or tuberculous dust could infect people who were in a condition to contract the disease, cleanliness and hygiene became of paramount importance both to sanatoria doctors and their architects. In order to minimise the risk of dried sputum causing infections, every effort was made to prevent dust accumulating on surfaces or in corners, and to exploit the germicidal property of sunlight. Cleanliness became the first line of defence against the disease, and sunlit buildings became fashionable. The dark, cluttered interiors which had been so popular with the Victorians and Edwardians were no longer considered hygienic. Instead the sunlit, airy, austere wards of the tuberculosis sanatorium became the ideal.

In the modern home furnishings, fabrics and fittings were arranged so that dust could be removed easily. Carpets were taken up and replaced by parquet floors and linoleum. Picture rails, pelmets, and ornate mouldings were taken down. Walls were decorated with washable paint and tiles rather than wallpaper which, when damp, was found to be an ideal medium on which to cultivate bacteria. Venetian blinds were adopted as an alternative to curtains, as they could be wiped clean of dust and adjusted to admit sunlight. In addition to its bactericidal effect, sunlight came to be valued for its capacity to promote cleanliness, as it enabled dirt and dust to be perceived more readily. Architects were encouraged to get sunlight into their buildings, and a new solar architecture emerged. It emphasized health and hygiene and became what we now know as modern architecture. Many of the leading figures of the Modern Movement were involved in sanatorium design and it is not altogether surprising that the 'sanatorium aesthetic' informed their designs for homes and offices.

However, as living standards began to improve, and antibiotics became available, the incidence of tuberculosis, scarlet fever, rheumatic fever and other infectious diseases declined. Consequently, hygiene, health and sunlight penetration ceased to be priorities for designers. The sunlit, well-ventilated offices and public buildings that were popular at the beginning of the 20th century fell out of favour. Deep-plan designs, which relied on efficient artificial lighting and excluded the sun, became popular with developers, if not occupants. When solar architecture was eventually reintroduced during the 1970s, it was for the purposes of energy conservation rather than health. By this time there were few incentives for designers and planners to create sunlit spaces other than to save energy, as sunlight was no longer considered therapeutic.

Although solar-heated buildings were shown to work well in the UK, energy efficiency was often achieved by imposing strict controls on internal conditions and excluding the influence of the external environment as much as possible. This is exactly the opposite of the approach recommended by Vitruvius and, not surprisingly, there is evidence that energy savings were made at the expense of the health of the people who worked in them.

Much of the current research on buildings and health is concerned with the so-called sick building syndrome found amongst office workers in the form of a range of recurrent symptoms such as headaches, lethargy, a dry throat, irritation to eyes and nose, and nausea. The causes of this syndrome have been notoriously difficult to identify and there are those who argue that it may have more to do with job satisfaction, or the lack of it, rather than bricks and mortar. The same cannot be said about the potentially far more serious threat to the health of a building's occupants posed by drug-resistant bacteria. As we have already seen, strains of tuberculosis are emerging which are resistant to antibiotics, and there are a number of other bacteria giving serious cause for concern.

If some of the more pessimistic warnings about drug-resistance are accurate we may have to introduce rather more air and light into our dwellings than we do at present, and make sure they are thoroughly clean. In these circumstances, air-conditioned, mechanically ventilated, open-plan offices, with their smoked-glass windows and artificial lighting, may not provide a particularly healthy environment. For one thing, fresh air is often in very short supply in buildings of this type: sometimes less than a fifth of the air is actually taken from outside, the rest being re-circulated. This would have been a dangerous practice during the pre-antibiotic era when major infectious diseases were commonplace.

Tuberculosis can certainly be passed from one person to another via ventilation systems. One famous outbreak, which occurred aboard a US naval vessel, the *USS Richard E Byrd,* illustrates the point. The air within the warship was fully re-circulated, which meant that there was little or no dilution of any infectious particles in the air. Someone with an undiagnosed case of tuberculosis was on board the ship for several months, during which time nearly half the crew became infected. The investigators brought in to study this outbreak concluded that direct personal contact played no part in the transmission of the tuberculosis, and that it had spread via the ship's mechanical ventilation system. More recently, the disease has been passed between passengers on long-haul commercial aircraft, but there is no clear evidence that tuberculosis bacteria have been transmitted via aircraft ventilation systems.

Since the 1950s much more emphasis has been placed on creating a 'comfortable' environment for building occupants than on promoting their wellbeing. But there is a great deal of difference between a comfortable atmosphere and a healthy one. So, before we get to a few of the practicalities of getting sunlight in and around buildings, it may be as well to learn what a healthy indoor environment actually is, and just how important it is to try to recreate outdoor conditions indoors. To this end we shall briefly examine the work of a scientist who was one of the great pioneers in the field of indoor health and who (it may come as no surprise to learn) was also a leading authority on the effects of sunlight and fresh air on the human body.

SIR LEONARD HILL: COMFORT OR HEALTH?

Sir Leonard Erskine Hill (1866–1952) was one of the most eminent physiologists of his generation. As director of the Department of Applied Physiology at the National Institute for Medical Research from 1914 to 1933, he carried out an extensive study of open air treatment and sunlight therapy, in which he worked closely with leading heliotherapists, including Sir Henry Gauvain. It was Leonard Hill who showed that open-air conditions speeded up the body's metabolic rate. He was also one of the first scientists to identify the factors that produce healthy conditions in buildings. Significantly, the recommendations put forward by Professor Hill on health and hygiene in buildings are very much at odds with conditions in today's houses, offices and hospitals, many of which are designed to produce a monotonous, over-warm, still atmosphere he strongly advised against.

Leonard Hill was born in Tottenham on the 2nd of June 1866. He graduated in medicine from University College London in 1889 and was awarded the degree of M.B. from the University of London the following year. After a period as a house surgeon, he returned to University College to pursue what was to be a long and distinguished career in physiology. Professor Hill believed that the inadequate ventilation and stagnant heating of dwellings and places of work, compounded with their occupants wearing too much clothing, overeating and taking too little exercise posed a significant threat to their health. He concluded from many years of detailed research that a warm, humid indoor environment was harmful

134

because it slowed down the body's metabolism, and that a sedentary life in too confined an atmosphere was a contributory cause of tuberculosis and other diseases. The design recommendations he put forward were intended to promote the wellbeing of the occupants and reduce their susceptibility to illness.

First and foremost he considered that cool conditions favoured bodily vigour and mental activity: a warm, humid indoor environment reduced the body's capacity to produce heat, which in turn lessened the appetite, depth of breathing, muscular tone and vigour of circulation, encouraging relaxation and sleep. In the course of his investigations Sir Leonard found that in many badly ventilated rooms the occupants' heads were too warm and their feet too cold, because floor temperatures were much lower than those at head level. He became convinced that conditions within a building should be as close as possible to ideal outdoor conditions which he defined in his book *Sunshine and Open-Air* in 1925 as follows:

> *The ideal method of warming and ventilating rooms would give*
> *radiant heat, a warm floor, and agreeable movement of cool air*
> *— the conditions of a sunny spring day out of doors.*

He firmly believed that the radiant heat of an open fire and the ventilation provided by its chimney, and by an open window when necessary, was the most healthy form of heating in the damp British climate; the radiant energy of the fire was particularly important as it made up for the absence of sunlight. In another book, *Health and Environment* published in 1925, Sir Leonard Hill anticipated gas-fired central heating. While recognizing its benefits in terms of energy efficiency and cleanliness, had strong reservations on health grounds:

> *Undoubtedly centralized heating would effect great economy of*
> *fuel and prevent smoke. Each house could be supplied with hot*
> *water and radiators from a central station. Cooking and fires for*
> *radiant heat could be supplied by gas. Nevertheless centralized*
> *heating produces a monotonous over-warm still atmosphere*
> *which will not promote health in people who have no*
> *opportunity for open-air exercise and who do not recognize the*
> *need for such.*

He believed that the human body required the stimulus of changing conditions if it was to prosper, and that a monotonous indoor environment was to be avoided. It is worth pointing out that Sir Leonard practised what he preached. He was a great believer in the saying 'Early to bed, early to rise' and for many years it was his daily habit, in all weathers, to take an early morning swim in a pond near his home. At the age of 85 he was still walking four miles a day. As one of his former colleagues put it in an obituary in the *British Medical Journal*:

> *The appearance of Leonard Hill as well as his words preached the gospel of sunshine and the open air. He seemed always to suggest in his person the peak of physical wellbeing.*

Incidentally, Sir Leonard was strongly of the opinion that the open-air treatment of tuberculosis should be based on sound physiological principles and not on blind belief in the virtues of 'fresh air'. This meant that patients should not be chilled and made miserable by the treatment — a sign that their capacity to generate internal heat had been exceeded. His extensive researches into the effects of open-air treatment and sunlight were motivated by the need to establish exactly how these conditions affect the human body. They may also have been influenced by the fact that he twice contracted pulmonary tuberculosis and recovered on both occasions. One of his sons also succumbed to the disease while on military service during the First World War and nearly died of it.

During his research Sir Leonard observed that people in outdoor occupations were free from 'colds' whatever exposure to extremes of temperature they underwent, for example, sailors on long voyages, lighthouse keepers and Arctic explorers. So, as far as he was concerned, the increase in respiratory disease which happens every winter was not due to lower temperatures out of doors, but to cold weather driving people indoors into stuffy, overheated rooms. He held that in these conditions the rate of infection was intensified and health weakened by heat stagnation, a lowered metabolism, and lack of sunlight.

For more than a century advocates of radiant heating have argued that it is healthier and more natural than warm-air heating, although this is still disputed. Radiant heating acts directly on the body and surrounding surfaces, creating comfortable conditions at lower air temperatures than would be the case with a warm-air system. The latter heats and circulates air which warms indirectly. Higher ambient temperatures are needed to achieve comparable comfort levels and one consequence of this, as Sir Leonard Hill discovered in the 1920s, is that the mucous membranes in the nose dry out, which increases susceptibility to infection. Also, because warm-air systems rely on air movement to transfer heat from the source to the occupants, they also move dust about which, again, increases the risk of infection and allergy.

What is striking about Professor Hill's findings on indoor health, if you can bear a little more historical background, is that they are almost identical to those Florence Nightingale placed before hospital designers in 1863 in her *Notes on Hospitals*. To Florence Nightingale, hospital buildings were central to the healing process as places where the sick would be restored to health as quickly and effectively as possible under the direct supervision of trained nursing staff. To create this healing environment a number of conditions had to be satisfied and, as she observed in *Notes on Hospitals*, they could only be satisfied by a competent hospital architect:

> *No ward is in any sense a good ward in which the sick are not*
> *at all times supplied with pure air, light and a due temperature.*
> *These are the results to be obtained from hospital architecture*
> *and not external design or appearance. Again, no one of these*
> *elements need be sacrificed in seeking to obtain the other.*
> *Anyone who feels himself in difficulty in realizing all three may*
> *rest satisfied that hospital architecture is not his vocation.*

She had learned some very harsh lessons about hygiene in hospitals shortly before this was written, and was keen to pass on the benefits of her experience to future generations. At the time of the Crimean War Florence Nightingale, in common with leading figures in the medical profession, had attached little importance to ventilation or sanitation. So sick men were packed together in the Scutari Barracks Hospital in what was an un-ventilated building on top of broken sewers. It was not until the end of the war that Miss Nightingale found out, to her horror, that the insanitary conditions within the hospitals she supervised in the Crimea had caused the deaths from sickness of 16,000 young men, while fewer than 2,600 had died in battle and 1,800 of their wounds. What made matters worse was that she had insisted to the Commander-In-Chief, Lord Raglan, that soldiers were sent to Scutari instead of staying at field hospitals near the front, where they would have had a much better chance of survival. As Hugh Small reveals in his recent investigation of this disaster, far from being the Angel of Mercy of popular myth, Florence Nightingale had unwittingly been an Angel of Death presiding over the loss of an entire army. This discovery, and her reluctant participation in the official cover-up which followed, brought on a complete breakdown which left her bedridden for many years.

Miss Nightingale dedicated the rest of her life to public health reforms. These included improving both sanitation and hospital design. One of the things that distinguishes her from some of the leading medical theorists of her day is that she became convinced of the revolutionary idea that fatal diseases could be caught from contaminated air: the so-called 'zymotic' theory of infection. This was very much at odds with the conventional thinking of the time which held that fatal diseases could only be spread by direct physical contact, and were caused by over work, lack of exercise, malnutrition or a 'broken constitution'. Armed with the 'zymotic' theory Miss Nightingale was able to explain why diseases spread in overcrowded conditions and how to design hospital wards to prevent this happening.

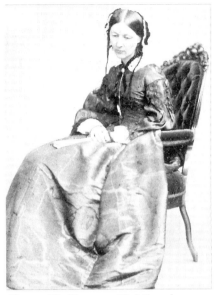

Figure 20: Florence Nightingale, an early advocate of sunlit wards

THE NIGHTINGALE WARD

Florence Nightingale became an advocate of 'pavilion plan' hospitals which consisted of single-storey ward blocks placed parallel to each other and joined by a corridor. Each of her pavilions was about 120 feet long by 30 feet wide and could accommodate some thirty beds. In terms of their overall dimensions the wards were designed to be large enough to be run by one head nurse, without being too large to ventilate by natural means. In part, pavilion wards were a development of Miss Nightingale's ideas on nursing which emphasized the need for someone to keep a very close eye on the staff and the patients at all times. To this end the wards were arranged so that the head nurse's room was next to the only entrance — and she had a window overlooking the whole ward. But one of the most important features that distinguished pavilion wards from other designs of the period was extensive glazing on both sides, with a minimum of one large window to every two beds. This meant that the wards could be cross-ventilated and admit sufficient fresh air and sunlight to stop hospital infections occurring. Together with her nursing philosophy, it was Florence Nightingale's belief in the zymotic theory which provided the rationale for such features. Her single-storey pavilion wards were designed to disperse contaminated air and prevent infections spreading from one part of the hospital to another.

THE FIREPLACE AND THE CHIMNEY

A large amount of fresh air was required to dilute and carry away the 'noxious emanations' of the sick and stop cross-infection, and the air within the wards had to be as fresh as it was outside. This could not be achieved by mechanical means as, in her opinion, no system of artificial ventilation could supply air which was sufficiently fresh. For one thing, there was no guarantee that the incoming air would not mix with the vitiated air. She insisted on natural ventilation not only because of her belief in the zymotic theory, but also because she believed that exposure to fresh air had therapeutic properties. So, for Florence Nightingale, natural ventilation and open fireplaces were the only suitable means of renewing and warming the air in hospitals. An open fireplace supplied radiant heat and its chimney was indispensable as a ventilating shaft. Radiant heat was natural; air heated by metal surfaces was to be avoided, particularly if it was supplied by the ventilation system. As she put it in *Notes on Hospitals:*

> *To shut your patients tight in artificially warmed air is to bake them in a slow oven.*

Miss Nightingale felt that if a hospital had to be ventilated artificially, it was because the original construction was defective in some way. Warm-air heating was not in accordance with 'Nature's Way' of providing fresh air, as it kept patients at one fixed temperature, day and night, during all the time they were in hospital. Variations of weather, temperature and season were important factors in the maintenance of health in healthy people, so the same should apply to the sick: patients needed to be exposed to the same continual changes in temperature and humidity that were occurring outdoors and so, weather permitting, the windows of every sick ward were to be kept open. These were effectively the open air conditions advocated by Dr George Bodington for the treatment of tuberculosis in his essay of 1840, except that Miss Nightingale was even more forthright in her views than he had been:

> *'Catching cold' in bed follows the same law as 'catching cold'
> when up. If the atmosphere is foul, and the lungs and skin
> cannot therefore relieve the system, then a draught upon the
> patient may give him cold. But this is the fault of the foul air,
> not the fresh. In the wooden huts before Sebastopol, with their
> pervious walls and open ridge ventilators, in which the patients*

said they 'would get less snow if they were outside', such a
thing as 'catching cold' was never heard of. The patients were
well covered with blankets, and all the better for the cold air.

As Florence Nightingale held that most infectious diseases were zymotic in origin, her views on health in buildings came to be regarded as unscientific and invalid. It has been argued that the discovery of germs and the benefits of antisepsis and asepsis left pavilion hospitals with no clinical advantages, or disadvantages, over other types. Almost as soon as the first Nightingale wards were being built it was alleged that they were no healthier than other ward designs and that they were expensive to build, administer and maintain. What should be borne in mind is that then, as now, the medical profession was rather more interested in improving public health by attacking specific diseases than in addressing the underlying conditions which caused them. Miss Nightingale had taken the opposite approach and tried to tackle infectious diseases in a way which would have found favour with Vitruvius and other engineers. In taking this 'engineering approach' she faced considerable resistance from the medical establishment to her campaign for sanitary reform and cleanliness in hospitals. To be fair, her design recommendations do owe a great deal to other hospital reformers who were medical men. But she eventually came to the conclusion that doctors and hospitals were detrimental to people's health and looked forward to a time when hospitals would no longer be needed. Be that as it may, some of the design principles described in her *Notes on Hospitals* were still being recommended by the Royal Institute of British Architects in their report *The Orientation of Buildings* in 1933, seventy years after they were first formulated:

> *It is gratifying to note that some architects are at last, although*
> *half a century too late, beginning to take advantage of Florence*
> *Nightingale's common sense…*

The environment within Nightingale wards was almost identical to that of the 'open-air' tuberculosis sanatoria which became popular in the 1920s and 30s. Like her wards, sanatoria buildings were in themselves instruments of cure, and the designs adopted for some of the better sanatoria were similar in many respects to the pavilion plan. In both cases fresh air was considered to have therapeutic properties and the buildings were designed to supply an abundance of it.

INDOOR HEALTH TODAY

It is quite striking how the indoor environment of the modern hospital departs from the principles set out by Florence Nightingale and Sir Leonard Hill. Nightingale wards are still in use today, but are heated and ventilated very differently from the way Miss Nightingale said they should be. There are, of course, good reasons for this. Medical practice has changed out of all recognition. Cold, fresh air is no longer considered to be therapeutic for hospital patients or, for that matter, anyone else. The diseases being treated now are very different from those of fifty or a hundred years ago. In wards where patients with cancer, heart disease, strokes, asthma and fractured hips now reside, there would once have been the victims of rheumatic fever, scarlet fever, typhoid fever, pneumonia, septicaemia, and a host of other infectious diseases. Patients in modern wards and, for that matter, the nursing staff, are used to much higher levels of comfort than their ancestors and they demand it.

Given a choice, human beings tend to opt for short-term comfort and turn a blind eye to the longer-term effects of their actions on their health. This is as true of the indoor environment we choose for ourselves as it is of own diet, recreational drugs and sedentary lifestyle. But for those of us who can resist these temptations, or have an overwhelming desire to open the windows of over-heated hospital wards whenever we are in them, Florence Nightingale's and Sir Leonard Hill's findings may be of more than passing interest.

If we want to be healthy indoors in the longer term, and are prepared to take some of these findings to heart, we may have to create as closely as possible *'the conditions of a sunny spring day out of doors'*. In the northern-European climate the solar-heated homes of the type Vitruvius described two thousand years ago come as close to this ideal as any. With this approach the direct radiant heat of the sun is stored in the building fabric and then re-radiated to the occupants later in the day when it is required. The internal environment is allowed to follow and modify external conditions rather than being held within closely defined limits. During overcast periods solar gains can be supplemented with radiant heat from an underfloor heating system. The Romans developed 'hypocausts' for their villas, passing heated air under the floors and walls to create radiant internal surfaces.

To get solar buildings to work properly there must be enough of the right material in the right place to absorb the incoming sunlight. Internal surfaces must provide effective thermal storage, and concrete floors, ceramic tiles and masonry walls are particularly suitable materials for this. The choice of internal finishes and fabrics also has a direct bearing on the effectiveness of the solar-heating strategy. After all, there is little point in putting in materials which store solar heat only to cover them over with fitted carpets that prevent the sunlight getting through. It may be more than just coincidence that the sort of interior best suited to keeping down dust and toxicity in dwellings is very similar to that needed to make the best use of radiant energy from the sun.

SUNLIGHT OUTDOORS

From the point of view of physical safety there is a great deal to be said for having the entrance to a building facing southeast or, at least, facing the direction of sunrise during the winter months. If there is no overshadowing from adjacent buildings or trees, the sun will melt snow and ice on paths and steps during the early part of the day. This reduces the risk of falls and other accidents caused by slippery surfaces which account for a significant number of admissions to Accident and Emergency units during the winter months, particularly amongst the elderly.

Sunlight on the exterior of buildings can also have a positive effect on the health of the people inside them. The walls of brick and concrete buildings absorb a large amount of moisture when it rains. This moisture dries out quickly on walls that get the sun and wind on them, otherwise it is retained for long periods. Damp wall surfaces which are not sunlit favour the growth of moulds and fungi. This can be very unhealthy, as the spores from these growths can find their way indoors, to be inhaled by the occupants. One way to prevent this is to make sure that the exterior of a building gets sunlight on it for as much of the year as possible. This means that close attention should be paid at the design stage to its orientation, as the positioning of a building affects the amount of sunlight it gets on its exterior. If it is set squarely with the cardinal points of the compass and faces due south, it will get very little sun at the back for almost half of the year. However, if it faces south east or south west, the walls will be sunlit through each season.

At a latitude of 51.5 degrees, that of London, a wall that faces due north gets no sun for six months of the year, but by June it enjoys over half an hour more possible sunshine than a wall facing northeast or northwest. Another rather odd fact is that a wall facing due south enjoys about 2 hours and 40 minutes more possible sunshine per day at the equinoxes than it does at midsummer. But at midsummer, the sun shines upon a southwest or southeast wall for more than half

142

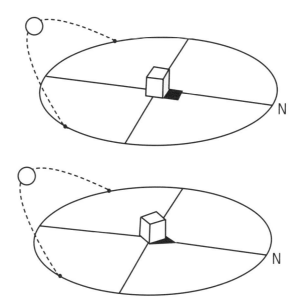

Figure 21: Orientation and sunlight: at northerly latitudes a building oriented due south will have a 'dark side' for several months each year

an hour longer than it does on a wall facing due south. These figures are based on the assumption that the sun shines from sunrise to sunset without interruption from clouds. However, over a year in Britain, there are on average about two hours of cloud for every hour of sunshine.

A building with a south-easterly orientation will get early morning sunlight into it for most of the year. Schools used to be designed with classrooms which faced southeast so that sunlight would warm, disinfect and make the rooms cheerful at the start of the school day. They had slightly projecting roof eaves over their windows which meant that in hot weather the sun would be sufficiently high up by the time children attended school to shine only a small distance into the rooms, and it was off the windows altogether later in the day. High-level windows on the northwest were sometimes used to allow summer sunshine into classrooms at the end of the school day. Sunlight therapy clinics were also arranged with this south-easterly orientation so that patients could take advantage of the rays of the early morning sun. In fact, schools and hospitals are rather unusual amongst building types in that they are often sited on open land, so their designers have an opportunity to orientate them carefully to make the interior spaces accessible to fresh air and winter sunlight.

THE ORIENTATION OF CITIES

Often it is the planning of a city which is the deciding factor in the amount of sunlight a building gets. If the streets and main thoroughfares are aligned with the cardinal points of the compass, there is every likelihood that everything else within the city is as well — including the buildings. The great American architect Frank Lloyd Wright commented on this in 1954 in his book *The Natural House:*

> Cities are commonly laid out north, south, east and west. This
> was just to save the surveyor trouble, I imagine. Anyway that
> happened without much thought for human beings compelled
> to build homes on those lines. This inevitably results in every
> house having a 'dark side'.

It is clear that the ancients appreciated the importance to health of the orientation of cities. The Greek philosopher Aristotle believed that the best orientation for cities was towards the east. Hippocrates was even more specific, and argued that cities that face the rising sun have the healthiest residents. Unfortunately, once a city is built there is little that can be done to alter its orientation. The same applies to the buildings in it, although windows and roof lights can be introduced to make more of sunlight and daylight.

INDOOR LIGHT

The sun is usually welcome in buildings as long as adequate precautions are taken to avoid visual or thermal discomfort. People generally don't like too much of it for too long: a great deal depends on their ability both to control the amount they let into a room and to change their position relative to it once it is in. The more freedom occupants have to alter these things, the less discomfort they experience. Rooms which face west are notoriously difficult to work in. Unless a great deal of care is given to shading and ventilation, glare and overheating will almost inevitably cause problems in the summer months, as anyone who has been confined in a west-facing office, kitchen or workshop during warm weather may know. Rooms with a northerly aspect, on the other hand, have long been favoured by artists because they provide steady lighting free of glare from the sun. It is for this reason that they are also popular with computer operatives who may struggle to see the screens of their VDUs in less favourable conditions. In recent years there has been a tendency to make north-facing windows in houses rather small so as to reduce heat loss. This can be something of a false economy because occupants then have to keep electric lighting on far longer than would have been the case if the windows had been made larger.

Changes are sometimes made to buildings that result in a reduction in the amount of sunlight and daylight penetration, and this can have a profound effect on the occupants. For example, during the Second World War the ground floor windows of many British hospitals were protected by brick blast-walls and had very poor daylight as a consequence. There was an outbreak of respiratory infection in the ground floor wards of one of these buildings — but not in the wards where the windows were unprotected. The difference was so marked that an investigation was undertaken by Dr Lawrence Garrod who was at that time Professor of Bacteriology at London University and bacteriologist to St. Bartholomew's Hospital.

He found that *haemolytic streptococci,* the bacteria which caused the infections, were far more numerous in dust samples taken from dark wards than in comparable specimens from wards with normal daylight where, close to unobstructed windows, even thick dust was consistently free from bacteria. Professor Garrod carried out a series of experiments which showed how important sunlight and daylight are in preventing the spread of infection. Like Dr Arthur Downes and Thomas Blunt before him, he found that direct sunlight had the strongest bactericidal effect. He also discovered that diffused light from a north window was capable of killing the bacteria, even though filtered through two layers of glass, while *streptococci* in dust kept in the dark survived for over six months. The results of Professor Garrod's investigation were reported in the *British Medical Journal* in 1944. They were:

> … *placed on record in order to draw attention to the possible importance of good natural illumination as a hygienic safeguard, and in the hope that they may lead to further study of this subject. Although good lighting is universally recognised as desirable, it has never, so far as I am aware, been insisted on as a prime necessity in wards for septic surgical cases. This study suggests that in such wards it has an important part to play, particularly if no special measures… are taken to prevent the atmospheric diffusion of dust.*

In fact, Florence Nightingale had insisted on this nearly a hundred years previously in her *Notes on Hospitals*. She is worth quoting at length on the subject of sunlit wards, if only to illustrate how easy it is to forget some of the most basic principles of healing and designing for health:

Direct sunlight, not only daylight, is necessary for speedy recovery, except, perhaps, in certain ophthalmic and a small number of other cases. Instances could be given, almost endless, where, in dark wards or in wards with a northern aspect, even when thoroughly warmed, or in wards with borrowed light, even when thoroughly ventilated, the sick could not by any means be made speedily to recover... All hospital buildings in this climate should be erected so that as great a surface as possible should receive direct sunlight — a rule which has been observed in several of our best hospitals, but, I am sorry to say, passed over in some of those most recently constructed. Window-blinds can always moderate the light of a light ward; but the gloom of a dark ward is irremediable... The escape of heat may be diminished by plate or double glass. But while we can generate warmth, we cannot generate daylight, or the purifying and curative effect of the sun's rays.

Coming up to date, there is a particularly striking example which illustrates the point. Modifications to the obstetric ward of a hospital in Papua New Guinea in the 1980s resulted in low levels of natural light which, in turn, caused an epidemic of jaundice amongst newborn infants in the ward. The architectural changes that produced the jaundice involved the extension of the roof overhangs above the windows. These extensions reduced the amount of indirect sunlight and daylight penetration to such an extent that the ward, which had formerly been bright and sunny, was dimly lit throughout the daytime. In these conditions the incidence of jaundice increased alarmingly from only 0.5 per cent to 17 per cent.

There are those who argue that jaundice in premature infants is actually caused by sunlight deprivation, and that it is the way in which obstetric wards and nurseries are designed that dictates the incidence of jaundice amongst the newborn. Measurements have shown that infants nursed in a sunlit ward can receive over 27,000 lux from the sun, while light levels in other comparable wards can be as low as 110 lux. So it seems that careful architectural planning could do a great deal to prevent a condition which is time-consuming for medical and nursing staff to manage and which can cause brain damage in newborn infants if treatment is delayed.

Again, high levels of illumination can be harmful for anyone who is unwell. In a neonatal clinic bright sunlight or artificial light might be damaging for the eyes of infants whose central retinas are immature at birth, and some form of shading should be provided for them. But certainly, if you have to spend any time in hospital, do try and get a bed in a sunlit ward. If the previous examples leave you unconvinced of the potential benefits, consider the results of a study published in the *Journal of the Royal Society of Medicine* in 1998, which looked at the records of over six hundred patients who were admitted to a cardiac intensive care unit after a first heart attack. Deaths were more frequent amongst patients who were put in sunless north-facing rooms than amongst patients in sunlit rooms. Also women patients, who generally do less well after a heart attack than men, were discharged earlier from sunny rooms than from the dull ones. The team that did this research was responsible for the study of depressed hospital patients described in Chapter 1. Not surprisingly, having discovered that sunny rooms were beneficent for clinically depressed patients, they began to consider the possible effects of sunny environments on other life-threatening conditions, and found that heart attack patients benefited from sunlight therapy, albeit accidentally. It will be interesting to see how research in this area develops and, more importantly, whether the findings persuade hospital architects to build more sunlit wards and nurseries than is the case at present.

Architects could do a great deal to reduce the amount of suffering and expense associated with degenerative bone diseases in the elderly, simply by providing sunlit balconies and verandahs. In 1984, residents at a home for the elderly in Auckland, New Zealand, took part in an experiment to see how much time they would have to spend in the sun each day to produce enough vitamin D to protect themselves against osteomalacia. Their average age was 80 years and, although mobile, they had to be helped with dressing and washing, and seldom went outdoors prior to taking part in this study. Sitting on the rest home's open verandah with their head and neck, forearms and lower legs exposed to the sun for only 30 minutes each day was all that was needed to achieve the required result, and this fitted easily into the daily routine of the residents and the nursing staff. The researchers who carried out this study, which was published in the journal *Age and Ageing,* concluded that sunning the frail elderly was an inexpensive, effective way to prevent osteomalacia without any of the risks of toxicity associated with taking oral supplements. They felt the benefits should be more widely appreciated by all personnel caring for the elderly, as well as by the elderly themselves, and that sheltered areas facing the sun need to be included in designs for rest homes.

One thing that the leading practitioners of heliotherapy had in common years ago was that they were actively involved in the design of hospitals and clinics. They had to be, because no one had built anything for sunlight therapy since the Fall of Rome. Sir Henry Gauvain became an expert on the design of wards for chronically ill patients, particularly adolescents and young adults who were recovering from surgical tuberculosis or were approaching convalescence. His experience in treating the long-term sick in balcony wards convinced him of the need for some accommodation of this type in every hospital and not just because of the opportunities it provided for sunlight exposure:

> ... if I may express my conviction, the most urgent and human need of most modern hospitals is the general lack of properly planned and protected balcony accommodation. Really to appreciate that need one should be a patient as well as a doctor. The advantage of getting into the open air, away from the sight, sounds and smells of the sick room, must be experienced to be understood and, in my opinion, this is a factor insufficiently recognised in practice.

Sir Henry wrote this in 1938, when it was quite common to have to stay in hospital for months at a time. Patients in modern hospitals are discharged much more quickly, but still run the risk of developing vitamin D insufficiency, or deficiency, while they are confined regardless of whether they are elderly or not. Hospitals should be built to allow patients who are strong enough to benefit from sunlight and fresh air to have access to them, as should homes for the elderly.

7

SUNLIGHT AND HEALTH
IN THE 21ST CENTURY

Our relationship with the sun is complex and attitudes to it have changed quite markedly throughout history. In 1903 the Nobel Prize for Medicine was awarded to a sunlight therapist and, in the years that followed, hospitals were built so that sunlight could be administered under medical supervision. But during the latter part of the 20th century the sun's rays have fallen from favour to such an extent that sunbathing is being actively discouraged. There can have been few more complete reversals in medical thinking.

Sunlight can harm, but there is a wealth of historical evidence which suggests that it can also heal and prevent chronic health problems. The physicians who used sunlight as a medicine during the first half of the 20th century knew sunlight therapy worked but were unable to explain why. They were, so to speak, working in the dark as there were few scientific theories that could adequately explain how sunlight speeded up the healing of wounds and reversed the damage caused by tuberculosis.

There is little scientific or, for that matter, historical evidence to support public health campaigns which recommend avoidance of the sun. There is no proof that sunlight causes melanoma, or that sunscreens prevent it. People who work indoors are at greater risk of developing the disease than those who work outdoors and melanoma tends to occur on the parts of the body less frequently exposed to sunlight such as the trunk and backs of the legs. In Europe, malignant melanoma is more common at higher latitudes where there is less sunlight, and a lifetime spent out in the sun decreases the risk of developing the disease. Lack of sunlight probably kills many thousands more people annually in this country than skin cancer. But, we need a much better understanding of the action of sunlight on the human body and the part it plays in preventing disease before we can be certain. More needs to be spent on finding out what sunlight does, and rather less on keeping us out of it.

Current research points increasingly to the important role played by vitamin D in the normal functioning of the body. Vitamin D is involved in the growth and maturation of cells and appears to have anti cancer properties. In laboratory experiments the biologically active form of vitamin D has been shown to inhibit the growth of malignant melanoma and other cancer cells. Vitamin D deficiency is implicated in a number of cancers and other major diseases. The action of sunlight on the skin is the natural way of producing vitamin D. So it is entirely plausible that the number of people who die each year of cancer of the breast, colon and prostate together with those who die from coronary heart disease, stroke and broken hips could be reduced by the adoption regular, moderate sunbathing.

Doubtless a great deal more will be discovered about the influence of vitamin D on the immune system in the years ahead, but what of sunlight itself? Why does sunlight exposure in childhood prevent multiple sclerosis developing in later life? How does our diet affect the way our skin responds to sunlight? What are the effects of sunscreen use on health in the longer term and what part is played by sunlight deprivation in the genesis of osteoporosis? Could the sun's rays be used to reverse the progress of the disease and others related to sunlight deprivation? Why is early morning sunlight so beneficial? We need answers to these and other questions but, unless there is a radical change in attitudes towards the sun amongst those who formulate public health policy, we are unlikely to get them.

It would certainly be very useful to know how common low vitamin D levels are across the whole population, and what exactly healthy levels of vitamin D are. Studies in Europe and North America suggest that insufficiency, if not deficiency could be much more common than is currently thought to be the case. Until this has been measured, recommendations as to the amount of sunlight exposure or dietary supplements needed to maintain adequate reserves are open to question. It is to be hoped that things become a little clearer in the not too distant future. Meanwhile, there seems little doubt that there is an epidemic of vitamin D deficiency among the older population. Those responsible for the care of the elderly, institutionalized or house-bound should be encouraged to take steps to ensure that their charges get enough sunlight, or enough supplements to prevent this occurring.

SUNLIGHT AND AN AGEING POPULATION

Demographic changes are under way which will have profound implications for the provision of healthcare for the elderly in the years ahead. More people are living longer, which means that the number with degenerative diseases is likely to increase significantly as we move into the 21st century. According to figures published by the World Health Organization, from 1990 to 1995, the population aged 65 and over increased by 14 per cent worldwide, and they predict an increase of 40 per cent in developed countries by the year 2020. Against this background, anything that helps older people to remain active, and free of disease and disability, should be given careful consideration by those who formulate public health policy. Regular, moderate exposure to the sun prevents osteomalacia in the elderly. For this reason alone older people should be encouraged, rather than discouraged, from going out in the sun.

One way to get a rather different perspective on the role of sunlight in preventing and curing diseases associated with ageing is to look to other traditions of healing. The physicians of ancient Greece and Rome used sunlight therapeutically, but the medicine of Hippocrates died out long ago. However, for those prepared to look further afield, both geographically and philosophically, there are other traditions which afford some useful insights. The Chinese have practised sunlight therapy since ancient times, and continue to do so. Their experience with sunlight, and the way they combine sunlight exposure with exercise are worthy of close examination, particularly in relation to the ageing process.

In a book entitled *Knocking at the Gate of Life and other Healing Exercises from China: The Official Exercise Book of the People's Republic of China*, which was published in the UK in 1985, sunlight therapy is recommended for a range of conditions including tuberculosis of the lungs, depression, heart disease, arthritis, rickets, and chronic enteritis or intestinal inflammation. This is entirely consistent with the practice of sunlight therapy in the west. However the Chinese use sunlight in other more subtle ways, and these seem to have some bearing on health in old age. To try and understand them it pays to know a little of the philosophy which underpins traditional Chinese medicine and exercise systems.

In traditional cultures older people are treated with dignity, as old age denotes wisdom. Chinese society has been based largely on respect for elders and for longevity. This interest in longevity has some of its roots in Taoism, a philosophy which has had a profound influence on Chinese culture. The early Taoists were alchemists who became keen students of the ageing process. Their investigations gave rise to the classical system of Chinese medicine and a number of other disciplines concerned with healing, such as exercise and diet therapy. Taoists held in high regard anyone who remained fit and healthy in old age. In doing so they reinforced the view that old age was something to aspire to. In contrast, western culture favours youth at the expense of the elderly, and positive role models for anyone over the age of about 60 are conspicuous by their absence. Western media tend to portray the elderly as dependent, decrepit or senile. The idea that a pensioner could possess levels of endurance or martial skills beyond those of a young adult is alien to our culture, but not to others.

In addition to respect for older members of society, the Chinese have a long and unbroken tradition of preventive medicine, and of paying close attention to the effects of natural cycles on health. They appear to have appreciated the beneficial effects of taking exercise in the early morning sun for hundreds, if not thousands, of years. The Chinese attach great importance to being outdoors at sunrise and exploit the health-giving properties of the early morning environment to the full. Over thousands of years they have developed and refined forms of exercise which, they believe, enable practitioners to accumulate 'biological energy' from the atmosphere. The most popular systems — such as t'ai chi and qigong — are used to this end in hospitals and by the population at large. The parks of Beijing, Shanghai and Hong Kong are full of older people practising at dawn each day. Exercise systems such as t'ai chi ch'uan are traditionally practised facing east, towards the rising sun. In India and elsewhere, practitioners of hatha yoga begin their early morning exercises with a 'Salute to the Sun', and Hippocrates wrote of the benefits of early morning walks in the winter months. So the findings of western heliotherapists, that early morning sunlight had the most beneficial effect on their patients, finds some support in traditional systems of healing.

Practitioners of t'ai chi and qigong argue that sunrise is the time of day with the greatest potential. The air is fresh and clear and full of 'goodness'. The chi in the air is more beneficial than at any other time because yang is increasing and yin energy is decreasing. Also, the organs of elimination — the lungs and large intestine — are at their most active just before dawn; so it is a good time to rid the body of stale energy and replenish it with early morning chi. To this end the Chinese have developed a vast array of what might be called 'open-air' exercises, and these form an integral part of their medical system. In his book *21st Century Medicine* Dr Julian Kenyon highlights the distinction between western and oriental medicine as follows:

152

The idea of biological energy is developed to a greater or lesser degree in different therapies, but probably finds its most sophisticated expression in Traditional Chinese Medicine where this energy is termed Chi… It comes as something of a surprise to realise that conventional medicine is the only medical system ever known to man which has no concept of biological energy.

As far as exercise is concerned, one of the most significant differences between East and West is directly related to ageing. Traditional Chinese exercise systems enable practitioners to increase their fitness and skills as they get older, and to cultivate their chi. For the most part, western systems dissipate chi, and the skill, fitness and stamina of sportsmen and women in the West decrease rapidly with advancing age. It might be useful, at this point, to examine some of the claims made for Chinese exercise, and find out why it differs from western exercise, and what the benefits of regular practice are.

First, a little of the history of the most popular system. According to legend, t'ai chi ch'uan, or taiji quan as it is written in romanized Chinese, was founded during the 13th century by a Taoist adept and martial arts expert called Zhang San Feng. The story goes that Zhang San Feng watched a battle between a crane and a snake, in which the snake outwitted the much bigger and stronger bird by skilfully evading each attack, and then retaliating with great speed and agility. He was so impressed with the flexibility and grace of the snake's movements that he decided to integrate them into a system of martial arts which also incorporated techniques of breath control, visualization and chi development. In the centuries that followed, t'ai chi developed into a formidable fighting system, and a means of refining the body's physiological and psychological processes in accordance with Taoist philosophical principles. Total concentration and mental quietness are required to perform t'ai chi ch'uan properly, and it combines the mind and body in a way that no western exercise does. In the West the mind has long been considered to be entirely separate from the body. Other cultures do not make this distinction; and at a practical level it is in the fields of medicine and exercise that this dichotomy is most apparent.

During the last few decades t'ai chi ch'uan has become very popular because of its health-giving attributes, and it is now practised by millions of people around the world. There is a growing body of evidence which shows that regular practice results in an improved general physical condition, and that the body's cardiovascular, respiratory and skeletal systems function more effectively. One of the many benefits of t'ai chi is that it improves balance. Loss of balance combined with poor general fitness and reduced flexibility can be as significant as low bone density in the occurrence of hip fractures. Falls are common among the elderly, often resulting in death or a general decline in health and mobility. A review of the benefits of t'ai chi practice published in the *Archives of Physical Medicine and Rehabilitation* in 1997 showed that there was a significant decrease in the onset of falls among elderly practitioners, together with a reduced fear of falling. Anyone who developed a drug which improved balance in this way, and was able to show that this reduced the costs of treating hip fractures and other fall-related injuries amongst the elderly, could look forward to a very comfortable retirement.

There is also evidence that t'ai chi is a very useful aid in the treatment of Parkinson's disease. This is a progressive neurological disorder with symptoms that include postural instability, trembling, slowness of movement, rigidity, depression and mental lethargy. Generally the incidence of hip fractures amongst sufferers of Parkinson's disease is high, and they also tend to be deficient in vitamin D with lower than average bone mass. Patients with the condition report that t'ai chi slows the decline of motor skills and mental ability normally associated with the disease. If it improves their balance as well, then the benefits of practising regularly could be very significant for anyone with the disease. Individuals with multiple sclerosis tend also to have low vitamin D levels and have a higher than average risk of hip fracture. As with Parkinson's disease, immobility and a deficient diet limit the amount of vitamin D available to them.

As a preventive measure at least, the Chinese approach to exercise seems to have a great deal to offer the increasing population of elderly and infirm in the West. Unfortunately there is no scientific evidence to back up claims as to the beneficial effects of exercise taken at dawn, other than it having therapeutic effect on patients with seasonal affective disorder. In the longer term, research may show that there are sound reasons for the traditional practice of gathering in parks and public spaces early morning to benefit from the subtle energies to which the Chinese attach such importance. After all, their long, unbroken tradition of folk medicine gives them a much more intimate and instinctive knowledge of what sunlight and fresh air does to the human body than we in the West have.

It is perhaps worth noting that Sir Henry Gauvain was unique amongst the leading heliotherapists of his day in that he did try to explain the action of the early morning sun in something approaching scientific terms. Like other heliotherapists, he observed over many years that morning light had the greatest therapeutic value and, in his opinion, this was because the 'light shock' of exposure to the early morning sun evoked a greater response in patients than exposure later in the day. Sir Henry developed this theme in what he called his 'theory of varying stimuli and varying response' which he presented to the Royal Society of Medicine in 1927. He argued that the naked body of a patient undergoing heliotherapy should be exposed to the open air under conditions that change seasonally and even daily and hourly. For him it was this constant change — which is more apparent in temperate climates than in the comparatively stable conditions found in many tropical regions — and the body's constant adaptation to this change that was the key to successful heliotherapy.

Although Sir Henry's ideas do not satisfactorily explain much that has been recorded about the effects of early morning sunlight or, indeed, heliotherapy in general, they do tie in to some extent with what is now known about seasonal affective disorder. There may well be more convincing theories for the health benefits of early morning light than the one proposed by Sir Henry Gauvain, and whether or not a satisfactory scientific explanation ever becomes available there seems little doubt that something rather profound goes on in the early hours of the day — clearly something other than the synthesis of vitamin D. The old saying 'Early to bed, early to rise' may have rather more to it than first meets the eye.

OZONE DEPLETION AND SUNSCREENS

While it is clear that the ozone layer is being depleted by the action of chemicals released into the atmosphere, there is as yet no sign of any long-term increase in UVB radiation in any of the World's more densely populated regions. The hole in the ozone layer may be a problem for workers in the Antarctic, but not for those of us a little nearer to the equator. The eye diseases, immune system disorders and environmental damage which were supposed to be upon us because of an increase in ultraviolet radiation have yet to materialise. Certainly, all of the available evidence shows that the increased incidence of skin cancer in the UK and elsewhere has not occurred because of ozone depletion.

So what is causing it? During the course of the 20th century the incidence of non-melanoma rates have increased dramatically and in industrialized countries this increase has been coincidental with the movement of populations from the land to take up work in offices and factories. We now spend a great deal of time indoors, consume fewer and fewer calories, and include a greater proportion of fat in our diets than ever before. Undoubtedly the influence of diet on cancer is profound and it may well be that nutrition, rather than sunlight, is at the very heart of the skin cancer problem.

When we do get sunlight, it is often when we are on holiday abroad after many months of being indoors and fully clothed. This means the slow, gradual pigmentation necessary to give the skin some natural protection from the intensity of Mediterranean or Caribbean sunshine does not take usually take place. In such circumstances, sudden bursts of strong solar radiation are not only unnatural but are also dangerous. While sunscreens can help prevent unpigmented skin from burning in these conditions, they should only ever be used as the very last line of defence. Skin that has not had time to build up its own protection against strong sunlight and a body that has not acclimatized are better protected by clothing, a hat and a long siesta.

One factor which may play a part in the genesis of skin cancer is the temperature of the surrounding environment. As we saw in chapter 3, the findings of a study published 1941 suggest that there may be a relationship between sunlight, ambient temperature and skin cancer, and that in places where the mean temperature is less than about 5.5°C, or 42°F, sunlight actually produces an immunity to it. From what is known from the work of Dr Auguste Rollier and other heliotherapists, the human body seems to react to sunlight very differently when trying to generate heat than when it is trying to lose it. Sunbathing in cool conditions seems to strengthen the immune system and stimulates the self-healing powers of the body. The reasons for this are not altogether clear, but it would certainly seem to be the safest approach to use when starting to sunbathe, unless you are very sensitive to cold conditions. Again, more research is urgently needed. The relationship between sunscreen use and malignant melanoma also needs to come under rather closer scrutiny than has been the case to date. This may meet with considerable opposition from those who promote there use, but there are respected scientists who question the advisability of using chemical sunscreens, and their concerns should be addressed.

Buildings, Bacteria and Sunlight

The number of people who die from skin cancer in the UK is about one tenth the number who die from infections caught in hospitals. Hospital infections now cause more deaths in the UK than either road traffic accidents or suicide. The emergence of drug-resistant bacteria is particularly worrying as it seems that blood poisoning, wound infections and pneumonia could soon be untreatable by every available antibiotic. The prospect of returning to the medicine of the pre-antibiotic era is daunting, yet this is what we may have to do if drugs fail and radical changes in medical practice are forced upon us. It is to be hoped that we never reach the stage where we have to rely as heavily on sunlight for the disinfection of wounds and the repair of bodies damaged by infectious diseases as our forebears did.

Certainly, if the problem cannot be resolved in the short term it will be important to find ways in which hospital buildings can be designed to prevent the spread of infection. Sunlit hospital wards have less bacteria in them than dark wards, and modern science is now showing that they provide a better environment for the treatment of clinically depressed patients and heart attack victims. Florence Nightingale said something to this effect in the 1860s, and a return to the standards of hygiene she insisted on would probably do a great deal to reduce the spread of infections in hospitals.

Getting sunlight into buildings to ensure a healthy indoor environment appears to have been particularly popular during periods in history when there was either overt sun-worship or the active use of sunlight as a therapeutic agent. At the present time, western culture is devoid of both sun-worship and sunlight therapy which helps to explain why we spend so much time in buildings that are not designed for sunlight. The Chinese have a well-established tradition of getting winter sunlight into their buildings, and this could be a manifestation of their concern to prevent disease. Similarly, the most famous architect of Imperial Rome, Vitruvius, stipulated that the bedrooms of houses and villas should face east to capture the early morning sun. Like his oriental counterparts he was concerned that dwellings should be arranged to secure the health of their occupants.

Vitruvius held that architects required a working knowledge of medicine. Given the health problems associated with living and working in contemporary buildings, perhaps building designers should undergo some form of medical training. Then again, perhaps we need an entirely new profession which embraces both disciplines. At least Vitruvius's clients would have got enough natural light into their properties to maintain their biological rhythms and emotional stability, which is more than can be said for many of us today.

As the human race evolved outdoors under the sun, and not indoors under strip-lights, it comes as no surprise that artificially lit environments can disturb the normal functioning of the body. Low light levels interfere with the natural production of melatonin so that too much of this hormone is secreted into the bloodstream in the daytime when we need to be alert, and too little at night when we need to sleep. Prolonged exposure to high levels of artificial light can put the body under stress, and there is also rather disturbing research which suggests that malignant melanoma could in some way be linked to exposure to fluorescent lighting. Of more immediate concern for those of us who follow the western lifestyle and spend most of our time behind glass, is that opportunities to benefit from the biologically active component of sunlight can be very limited.

While exposure to the sun can undoubtedly pose severe health risks, many of us may be compromising our health because we are deprived of it. The aim of this book has been to highlight some of the positive aspects of the sun, and to give some guidance on how to minimize the risks and maximize the benefits of exposure. Much remains unknown about the action of sunlight on the human body. By the same token, the causes of many of the major degenerative diseases which hold the western world in their grip are far from clear. Sunlight or, rather, sunlight deficiency may play a much greater role in the genesis of these diseases than is generally recognized. There is a substantial body of historical and contemporary evidence that suggests that moderate sunbathing could be rather more beneficial than we are currently led to believe. If you are convinced of this, proceed with caution and keep in mind those fateful words inscribed at the Temple of Apollo: *'All things in moderation . . . Know thyself.'*

REFERENCES

Chapter 1

Allen, R.M., and Cureton, T.K., 'Effect of Ultraviolet Radiation in Physical Fitness', *Arch Phys Med 26,* 1945, 641 – 644

Anon, Committee on the Medical Aspects of Food and Policy Department of Health Report on Nutrition and Bone Health: with Particular Reference to Calcium and Vitamin D, Department of Health Report on Health and Social Subjects No. 49, HMSO, 1991

Anon, Sunshine & Skin Cancer, Consensus Statement, UK Skin Cancer Prevention Working Party, 1997

Black, D., 'Does Sunlight Heal or Harm?', *The Health Consumer's Health and Wellness Report,* 3, 6, Tapestry Communications Inc., 1993

Beauchemin, K.M., and Hays, P., 'Sunny Rooms Expedite Recovery From Severe and Refractory Depressions', *J Affective Disorders,* 40, 1996, 49–51

Bock, J.S., and Boyette, M., *Stay Young the Melatonin Way,* Vermillion, London, 1995

Celsus, De Medicina (Trans. Spenser, W.G.), Heineman, London, MCMXXXV

Chel, V.G.M., Ooms, M.E., Popp Snuders, C., Pavel, S., Shothorst, A.A., Meulemans, C.C.E., et al., 'Ultraviolet Irradiation Corrects Vitamin D Deficiency and Suppresses Secondary Hyperparathyroidism in the Elederly', *J Bone Miner Res,* 13, 8, 1998, 1238–1242

Davey Smith, G., Neaton, J.D., Wentworth, D., et al., Mortality Differences Between Black and White Men in the USA: 'Contribution of Income and other Risk Factors among Men screened for the MRFIT Research Group. Multiple Risk Factor Intervention Trial', *Lancet,* 10, 1, 1051–1056

Dobbs, R.H., and Cremer, R.J., 'Phototherapy', *Arch Dis Child,* 50, 1975, 833–6

Darlington, J., 'Ultraviolet – the True Story', *Positive Health,* Oct./Nov., 1995

Donawho, C., and Wolf, P., 'Sunburn, Sunscreen and Melanoma', *Current Opinion in Oncology,* 8, 1996, 159–166

Downing, D., *Day Light Robbery,* Arrow Books, London, 1988

Dyer, A.R., Stamler, J., Berkson, D.M., et al., 'High Blood-Pressure: a Risk Factor for Cancer Mortality?', *J Natl Cancer Inst,* 77, 1, July 1986, 63–70

Eastwood, J., and Gorman, J., *Understanding Seasonal Affective Disorder,* Mind Publications, 1994

Eberlein Konig, B., Placzek, M., and Przybilla, B., 'Protective Effect Against Sunburn of Combined Systemic Ascorbic Acid (Vitamin C) and d-alpha-tocopherol (Vitamin E)', *J Am Acad Dermatol,* 38, 1, 1998, 45–8

Epstein, J.H., 'Effects of Beta-Carotene on UV-induced Cancer Formation in the Hairless Mouse', *Photochem Photobiol,* 25, 1977, 211

Goldbourt, U., Holtzman, E., Yaari, S., et al., 'Elevated Systolic Blood Pressure as a Predictor of Long-Term Cancer Mortality: Analysis by Site and Histological Subtype in 10,000 Middle-Aged and Elderly Men', *J Nat Cancer Inst,* 771, July 1986, 63–70

Guthrie, D., *A History of Medicine,* London, 1958

Hawkes, J., *Man and the Sun,* The Cresset Press, London, 1962

Holick, M.F., Matsuoka, L.Y., and Wortsman, J., 'Regular Use of Sunscreen on Vitamin D Levels', *Arch Dermatol,* 1995, 131,11, 1337–1339

Holick, M.F., 'The Photobiology of Vitamin D and its Consequences for Humans', *Ann New York Acad Sci,* 453, 1985, 1–13

Holick M.F., 'Vitamin D and Bone Health', *J Nutr,* 126, 4, 1996 Suppl, 1159S–64S

Holick, M.F., 'Vitamin D – New Horizons for the 21st Century', *Am J Clin Nutrition,* 60, 1994, 619–630

Kime, Z.R., *Sunlight Could Save Your Life,* World Health Publications, Penryn, California, 1980

Krause, R., Buhring, M., Hopfenmuller, W., Holick, M.F., and Sharma, A.M., 'Ultraviolet B and Blood Pressure', *Lancet,* 352, August 29th, 1998, 709–710

Lansdowne, A. T. and Provost, S. C., 'Vitamin D3 Enhances Mood in Healthy Subjects During Winter', *Psychopharmacology,* 135, 4, 1998, 319–323

Laurens, H., 'The Physiological Effects of Ultraviolet Radiation', *J Am Med Assn,* 111, 1939, 2385–2392

Liberman, J.I., *Light: Medicine of the Future,* Bear & Co., Santa Fe, 1991

Lohmeier, L., 'Let the Sun Shine In', *East West,* July 1986, 36–43

Mawer, E.B, *The Sunshine Vitamin: A Guide to Understanding the Prevention and Treatment of Vitamin D Deficiency,* Shire Osteoporosis Society, Hampshire, 1992

Partonen, T, 'Vitamin D and Serotonin in Winter', *Med Hypothesis,* 51, 3, 1998, 267–268

Reid, I.R., Gallagher, D.J. and Bogsworth, J., 'Prophylaxsis Against Vitamin D Deficiency in the Elderly by Regular Sunlight Exposure', *Age and Ageing,* 15, 1986, 35–40

Rosen, L.N., Targum, S.D., Terman, M., et al., 'Prevalence of Seasonal Affective Disorder at Four Latitudes', *Psychiatry Res,* 31, 2, 131–144

Rostand, R.G., 'Utraviolet Light May Contribute to Geographic and Racial Blood Pressure Differences', *Hypertension,* 1997 August 30:2 Pt 1, 150–6.

Rowe, D., *Breaking The Bonds,* Fontana, London, 1991

Smyth, A., *Seasonal Affective Disorder,* Thorsons, London, 1997

Sobel, D., *Longitude,* Fourth Estate, London, 1996

Weber, G.W., Prossinger, H., and Seidler, H., 'Height Depends on Month of Birth', *Nature,* 391, 1998, 754–755

Wirz-Justice et al., 'Natural Light Treatment of Seasonal Affective Disorder', *J Affective Disorders* 37, 1996, 109–120

Wurtman, R.J., 'The Effects of Light on Man and other Mammals', *Ann Rev Physiol,* 37, 1975, 467–483

Wurtman, R.J., 'The Pineal and Endocrine Function', *Hospital Practice,* January 1969, 32–37

Chapter 2

Abramov, I., 'Health Effects of Indoor Lighting: Discussion', *Ann New York Acad Sci,* 453, 1985, 365–370

Addison Jayne, W., *The Healing Gods of Ancient Civilizations,* University Books, New York, 1962

Anon., 'Sunscreen Protection Controversy Heats Up', *J Am Med Assn,* 265, 24, 1991, 3218–3220

Anon., 'Do Sunscreens Prevent Skin Cancer?' *Johns Hopkins Med Lett Health,* 4, June 10, 1998

Anon., 'Are Sunscreens a Cancer Smokescreen?', *East West,* January 1989, 40–43

REFERENCES

Ashwood-Smith, M.J., 'Possible Cancer Hazard associated with 5-methoxypsoralen in Suntan Preparations', *British Medical Journal*, 3 November 1979, 1144

Autier, P., Dore, J.F., Cattaruzza, M.S., et al., 'Sunscreen Use, Wearing Clothes, and Number of Nevi in 6- to 7-Year-Old Children', *J Nat Cancer Inst,* 90, 1998, 1873–80

Bailey, A., *The Caves of the Sun*, Jonathan Cape, London, 1997

Berwick, M., and Halpern, A., 'Melanoma Epidemiology', *Current Opinion in Oncology,* 1998, 9, 0178-0182 1989, 517–521

Bloom, B.R. and Murray, C.J.L., 'Tuberculosis: Commentary on a Re-emergent Killer,' *Science,* 257, 21 August 1992, 1054–1064

Coleman, V., *Bodypower*, European Medical Journals, Barnstaple, Devon, 1994

Dewan, E., 'Possibility of a Perfect Rhythm Method of Birth Control by Periodic Light Stimulation', *Am J Obst & Gynaec,* 99, 7, 1967, 1016–1019

Diffey, B. L., 'Sun Protection: Have We Gone Too Far?' *Brit J Dermatol,* 138, 1998, 562–563

Durie, B., 'Why Bother with a Suntan?', *New Scientist,* 14th August, 1990, 516–517

Eberlein Konig, B., Placzek, M., and Przybilla, B., 'Protective Effect Against Sunburn of Combined Systemic Ascorbic Acid (Vitamin C) and d-alpha-tocopherol (Vitamin E)' *J Am Acad Dermatol,* 38, 1, 1998, 45–8

Garland, C.F., Garland, F.C., and Gorham, E.D., 'Lack of Efficacy of Common Sunscreens in Melanoma Prevention', in *Epidemiology, Causes and Prevention of Skin Diseases,* (Eds. Grob, J.J., Stern, R. S., MacKie, R.M., and Weinstock, W.A.), Blackwell Science, Chapter 11, 152–159

Garland, C.F., Garland, F.C., and Gorham, E.D., 'Could Sunscreens Increase Melanoma Risk?', *Am J Public Health,* 82, 4, 1992, 614–615

Griggs, B., 'A Veritable Feast for the Eyes', *The Independent,* 9 October 1990, 17

Harding, J.J., 'Testing Time for the Sunlight Hypothesis of Cataract', *Current Opinion in Opthalmology,* 7, 1, 1996, 159–162

Harding, J.J., 'The Untenability of the Sunlight Hypothesis of Cataractogenesis', *Documenta Opthalmologica,* 88, 1995, 345–349

Hawk, J. L. M., 'Ultraviolet A Radiation: Staying Within the Pale', *British Medical Journal,* 302, 4th May 1991, 1036–1037

Hinds, M.W. 'Nonsolar Factors in the Etiology of Malignant Melanoma', *Nat Cancer Inst Monogr,* 1992, 62, 173–178

Huxley, A., *The Art of Seeing,* Flamingo, London, 1994

Larsen, H.R., 'Do Sunscreens Cause Cancer?' *J Alternative and Complementary Medicine*, 12, 1994, 17–19

Le Fanu, J., 'Sunbathing, 'skin cancer' and Sore Confusion', *The Sunday Telegraph,* Review, July 18, 1999, 4

Lieberman, B., 'Doomsday Deja Vu: Ozone Depletion's Lessons For Global Warming', Working Paper, The European Science and Environment Forum, Cambridge, November 1998

McGregor, J.M. and Young, A.R., 'Sunscreens, Suntans, and Skin Cancer', *British Medical Journal,* 312, 29th June, 1996, 1612–1613

Moan, J., and Dahlback, A., 'The Relationship Between Skin Cancers, Solar Radiation and Ozone Depletion', *Brit J Cancer,* 65, 1992, 916–921

Neer, R.M., 'Environmental Light: Effects on Vitamin D Synthesis and Calcium Metabolism in Humans', *Ann New York Acad Sci*, 453, 1985, 15–21

Nicholas, A., Phelps Brown, A, Harding, J. J. and Dewar, H., 'Nutrition Supplements and the Eye', *Eye*, 12, 1998, 127–133

Norman, A.W., 'Sunlight, Season, Skin Pigmentation, Vitamin D, and 25-hydroxyvitamin D: Integral Components of the Vitamin D Endocrine System', *Am J Clinical Nutr*, 67,6, June, 1998, 1108–10

Olcott, W. T., *Sun Lore of All Ages*, G.P. Putnam's Sons, London, 1914

Osler. W., *The Evolution of Modern Medicine*, Oxford University Press, 1922

Pearce, F., 'Ozone Hole Innocent of Chile's Ills', *New Scientist*, 21st August, 1993, 7

Prentice, A.M., and Jebb, S.A., 'Obesity in Britain: Gluttony or Sloth?' *British Medical Journal*, 311, 1995, 437–439

Rees, J. L., 'The Melanoma Epidemic: Reality and Artefact', *British Medical Journal*, 312, 20th January 1996, 137

Ridley, M., 'Taking the Sting out of the Sunshine Myth', *The Sunday Telegraph*, 3rd April, 1994

Roberts, L.K., and Beasley, D.G., 'Sunscreen Lotions Prevent Ultraviolet Radiation-Induced Suppression of Antitumor Immune Responses', *Int J Cancer*, 71,1, 1997, 94–102

Schauder, S., and Ippen, H., 'Contact and Photocontact Sensitivity to Sunscreens. Review of a 15-Year Experience and of the Literature', *Contact Dermatitis*, 37, 5 1997, 221–232

Schein, O.D., Vicencio, C., Müoz, B., et al., 'Ocular and Dermatologic Health Effects of Ultraviolet Radiation Exposure from the Ozone Hole in Southern Chile', *Am. J Public Health*, 85, 4, April 1995, 546–550

Singh, M., *The Sun in Myth and Art*, Thames and Hudson, London, 1993

Walter, S.D., Marrett, L.D., Shannon, H.S., et. al., 'The Association of Cutaneous Malignant Melanoma and Fluorescent Light Exposure', *Am J Epidemiol*, 135, 1992, 749–762

Wei, Q., 'Vitamin Supplementation and Reduced Risk of Basal Cell Carcinoma', *J Clin Epidemiol*, 47 , 1994, 829–836

Westerdahl, J., Olsson, H., Masback, A., et al., 'Is the Use of Sunscreens a Risk Factor for Malignant Melanoma?', *Melanoma Research*, 5, 1995, 59–65

Winstock et al., 'Controversies in the Role of Sunlight in the Pathogenesis of Malignant Melanoma', *Photochemistry and Photobiol*, 63, 1996, 4, 406–410

Zlotkin, S., 'Vitamin D Concentrations of Asian Children Living in England. Limited Vitamin D Intake and Use of Sunscreens', *British Medical Journal*, 318, 1999, 1417

Chapter 3

Acheson, E.D., Bachrach, C.A. and Wright, F.M., 'Some Comments on the Relationship of the Distribution of Multiple Sclerosis to Latitude, Solar Radiation and other Variables', *Acta Psychiatr Scand*, 35, Suppl 147, 1960, 132–147

Aiken, J.M. and Anderson, J.B., 'Seasonal Variations in Bone Mineral Content After the Menopause', *Nature*, 241, 5th January 1973, 59–60

Ainsleigh, H.G., 'Beneficial Effects of Sun Exposure on Cancer Mortality', *Preventive Medicine*, 22, 1993, 132–140

Anon, 'Vitamin D Supplement in Early Childhood and Risk for Type 1 (insulin dependent) Diabetes Mellitus. The EURODIAB Substudy 2 Study Group', *Diabetologica*, 42, 1, 1999, 51–54

Anon., 'Vitamin D Deficiency Deemed Widespread', *Tufts University Health & Nutrition Letter,* 16, 3, May 1998, 1 & 6

Anon., Cancer Research Campaign Factsheet, 1.1, CRC, London, 1994

Anon., Cancer Research Campaign Factsheet, 3.1, CRC, London, 1995

Anon., 'Cancers to Rise by Nearly 70%', News Release, Macmillan Cancer Relief, London, 25 June, 1997

Anon., *The World Health Report,* World Health Organization, Geneva, 1997

Apperley, F.L., 'The Relation of Solar Radiation to Cancer Mortality in North America', *Cancer Res,* 1, 1941, 191–195

Baron, Y.M., Brincat, M., Galea, R. and Baron, A.M., 'The Epidemiology of Osteoporosis in a Mediterranean Country', *Calcif Tissue Int,* 54 ,4, May 1994, 365–369

Bentham, G., 'Association Between Incidence of Non-Hodgkin's Lymphoma and Solar Ultraviolet Radiation in England and Wales', *British Medical Journal,* 4th May 1996, 312, 1128–1131

Bikle, D.D., 'Role of Vitamin D, its Metabolites, and Anologs in the Management of Osteoporosis', *Rheum Dis Clin North Am,* 20, 3, 1994, 759–775

Binet, A., and Kooh, S.W., 'Persistence of Vitamin D-Deficiency Rickets in Toronto in the 1990s', *Can J Public Health,* 87, 4, 227–230

Brook, O.G., Brown I.R.F., and Cleeve, H.J.W., 'Vitamin D Deficiency in Asian Immigrants', *British Medical Journal,* 21 July 1979, 206

Chamberlain, J., *Fighting Cancer,* Headline, London, 1997

Chapuy, M.C., et al., 'Prevalence of Vitamin D Insufficiency in an Adult Normal Population', *Osteoporosis Int,* 7, 5, 1997, 439–443

Chel, V.G.M., Ooms, M.E., Popp Snuders, C., Pavel, S., Shothorst, A.A., Meulemans, C.C.E., et al., 'Ultraviolet Irradiation Corrects Vitamin D Deficiency and Suppresses Secondary Hyperparathyroidism in the Elderly', *J Bone Miner Res,* 13, 8, 1998, 1238–1242

Compston, J.E., 'Vitamin D Deficiency: Time For Action', *British Medical Journal,* 317, 28th November 1998, 1466–1467

Cummings, S.R., Kelsey, J.L., Nevitt, M.C., and O'Dowd, K.J., 'Epidemiology of Osteoporosis and Osteoporotic Fractures', *Epidemiol Rev,* 7, 1985, 178–207

Davies, D.M., 'Calcium Metabolism in Healthy Men Deprived of Sunlight', *Ann New York Acad Sci,* 453, 1985, 21–27

Downing, D., *Day Light Robbery,* Arrow Books, London 1988

East, B.R., 'Mean Annual Hours of Sunshine and the Incidence of Dental Caries', *Am J Public Health,* 29, 1939, 777–780

Elwood, M.J. and Jopson, J., 'Melanoma and Sun Exposure: An Overview of Published Papers', *Int J Cancer,* 73, 1997, 198–203

Even-Paz, Z., and Shani, J., 'The Dead Sea and Psoriasis: Historical and Geographic Background', *Int J Dermatology,* 28, 1, 1989, 1–9

Freedman D.M., Zahm, S.H. and Dosemeci, M., 'Residential and Occupational Exposure to Sunlight and Mortality from Non-Hodgkins Lymphoma: Composite (Threefold) Case Control Study', *British Medical Journal,* 314 May 17 1997 1451–1455

Garland, F.C., Garland, C.F., Gorham, E.D, and Young, J.F., 'Geographic Variation in Breast Cancer Mortality in the United States: a Hypothesis Involving Exposure to Solar Radiation', *Prev Med,* 19, 1990, 614–622

Garland, C.F., and Garland, F.C., 'Does Sunlight and Vitamin D Reduce the Likelihood of Colon Cancer?', *Int J Epidemiol*, 9, 3, 1980, 227–231

Garland, F.C, and Garland, C.F., 'Occupational Sunlight Exposure and Melanoma in the U.S. Navy', *Archives of Environmental Health*, 45, 5, 1990, 261–267

Garland, C.F., Garland, F.C., and Gorham, E.D., 'Epidemiology of Cancer Risk and Vitamin D' in *Vitamin D: Molecular Biology, Physiology, and Clinical Applications*, (Ed. Holick, M.F.), Humana Press, New Jersey, 1999, Chapter 22, 375–391

Garland, F.C., Garland, C.F., and Gorham, E.D., 'Colon Cancer Parallels Rickets', in *Calcium, Vitamin D, and Prevention of Colon Cancer*, (Eds. Lipkin, M., Newmark, H.L., and Kelloff, G.) CRC Press, Boston, 1991, 81–111

Gibbs, D., 'Rickets and the Crippled Child: an Historical Perspective', *J Roy Soc Med*, 87, December 1994, 729–732

Gorham, E.D., Garland, C.F., and Garland, F.C., 'Acid Haze Air Pollution and Breast and Colon Cancer Mortality in 20 Canadian Cities', *Can J Public Health*, 80, 1989, 96–100

Grimes, D.S., Hindle, E., and Dyer, T. 'Sunlight, Cholesterol and Coronary Heart Disease', *Quarterly Journal of Medicine*, 89, 1996, 579–589

Gross, C., Stamey, T., Hancock, S. and Feldman, D., 'Treatment of Early Recurrent Prostate Cancer with 1,25-dihydroxyvitamin D3', *J Urol*, 159, 6, 2035–2039

Hanchette, C.L., and Schwartz, G.G., 'Geographic Patterns of Prostate Cancer Mortality', *Cancer*, 1992, 70, 2861–9

Harris, S.S., and Dawson-Hughes, B., 'Seasonal Changes in 25-hydroxyvitamin D Concentrations of Young American Black and White Women', *Am J Clin Nutr*, 67, 1998, 1232–1236

Hawk, J.L.M., 'Ultraviolet A Radiation: Staying Within the Pale', *British Medical Journal*, 302, 4th May 1991, 1036–1037

Hays C.E., Cantorna M.T. and DeLuca, H.F., 'Vitamin D and Multiple Sclerosis', *Proc Soc Exp Biol Med*, 1997 Oct., 216:1, 21–27

Herodotus, *The Histories*, (Trans. de Sélincourt, A.), Penguin Books, London, 1972

Horio, T., 'Skin Disorders that Improve by Exposure to Sunlight', *Clin Dermatology*, 16,1, 1998, 59–65

Hutter, C.D. and Laing, P., 'Multiple Sclerosis, Sunlight, Diet, Immunology and Aetiology', *Med Hypothesis*, 46, 2, Feb 1996, 67–74

Illman, J., 'Cold Comfort', *The Guardian*, July 23rd 1996, 15

Jacobsen, S.J., Goldberg, J., Miles, T.P., Brody, J.A., Stiers, W., and Rimm A.A., 'Seasonal Variation in the Incidence of Hip Fracture among White Persons Aged 65 Years and Older in the United States', *Am J Epidemiol*, 133, 1991, 996–1004

Jacobson, B., Smith, A. and Whitehead, M., (Eds.) *The Nation's Health: A Strategy for the 1990s*, The King's Fund Centre, London, 1991

Johnson, J.R., et al., 'The Effect of Carbon-Arc Radiation on Blood Pressure and Cardiac Output', *Am J Physiol*, 114, 1935, 594–602

Khaw, T.K., Sneyd, M.J., and Compston, J., 'Bone Density Parathyroid Hormone and 25-hydroxyvitamin D Concentrations in Middle Age Women', *British Medical Journal*, 305, 1992, 273–7

Kime, Z.R., *Sunlight Could Save Your Life*, World Health Publications, Penryn, California, 1980

Kodicek, E., 'The Story of Vitamin D: From Vitamin to Hormone', *Lancet*, i 1974, 325–329

Kushelevsky, A.P., et al., 'Safety of Solar Phototherapy at the Dead Sea', *J Am Acad Dermatol*, Vol 38, No 3, 1998, 447–452

164

References

Lawson, D.E.M, Paul, A.P, and Black, A.E., et al., 'Relative Contributions of Diet and Sunlight to Vitamin D State in the Elderly', *British Medical Journal*, August 4th, 1979, 303–305

Loomis, W.F., 'Rickets', *Scientific American,* 223, 1970, 77–91

Malabanan, A., Veronikis, I.E., and Holick, M.F., 'Redefining Vitamin D Insufficiency', *Lancet*, 351, March 14, 1998, 805–806

Mays, K., *Osteoporosis,* Thorsons, London, 1991

McBeath, E.C., and Zuker, T.F., 'The Role of Vitamin D in the Control of Dental Caries in Children', *Journal of Nutrition,* 15, 1938, 547

McIlwain, H.M., Bruce, D.F., Silverfield, J.C., et al., *Winning with Osteoporosis,* John Wiley and Sons, New York, 1993

McMichael, A. J., and Hall, A. J., 'Does Immunosuppressive Ultraviolet Radiation Explain the Latitude Gradient for Multiple Sclerosis?' *Epidemiology,* 8, 6, Nov., 1997, 642–645

Mozolowski, W., 'Jedrzej Sniadecki (1768–1883) on the Cure of Rickets', *Nature*, 143, 1939, 121

Ness, A. R., Frankel, S. J., et al., 'Are We Really Dying for a Tan?', *British Medical Journal*, 319, 1999, 114–116

Nordin, B.E., 'Calcium and Osteoporosis', *Nutrition*, 13, 7–8, 1997, 664–86

Ott, J.N., *Health and Light,* Pocket Books, New York, 1973

Peller, S., Skin Irradiation and Cancer in the US Navy', *American Journal of Medical Science,* 194, 1937, 326–333

Riggs, B.L., 'The Worldwide Problem of Osteoporosis: Insights afforded by Epidemiology', *Bone,* 17 (5 Suppl:) Nov. 1995, 505S–511S

Rosen, L.N., Livingstone, I.R. and Rosenthal, N.E., 'Multiple Sclerosis and Latitude: A New Perspective on an Old Association', *Med Hypothesis*, 36, 4, 1991, 376–378

Schneider Lefkowitz, E. and Garland, C.F. 'Sunlight, Vitamin D, and Ovarian Cancer Mortality Rates in US women', *Int J Epidemiol*, 23, 6, 1994, 1133–1136

Schreus, H.T., 'Karl Linser's Discovery of Heliotherapy for Mycosis Fungoides', *Dermatol Wochenschr,* 151, 37, 1965, 1069–1074

Schwartz, G.G., and Hulka, B.S., Is Vitamin D Deficiency a Risk Factor for Prostate Cancer? (Hypothesis)', *Anticancer Research,* 10, 1990, 1307–1312

Stockton, D., *Report of Cancer Incidence and Prevalence Projections,* Macmillan Cancer Relief, London, June 1997

Studzinski, G.P., and Moore, D.C., 'Sunlight – Can it Prevent as well as Cause Cancer?', *Cancer Research*, 55, 1995, September 15, 4014–4022

Thomas, M.K., Lloyd-Jones, D.M., et al., 'Hypovitaminosis D in Medical Inpatients', *New Eng J Med,* 338, 1998, 777–783

Tipple, H. and Engst, R., 'Mycosis Fungoides: Results of Helioclimate Therapy in the High Alps', *Hautarzt,* 37, August, 1986, 450–453

Utiger, R. D., 'The Need for More Vitamin D', *N Eng J Med,* 338, 1998, 828–829

Van Der Wielen, R.P.J., Lowick, M.R.H., Van Den Berg, H., et al., 'Serum Vitamin D Concentrations Among Elderly People in Europe', *Lancet*, 346, July 22, 1995, 207–210

Veith, R., Vitamin D Supplementation, 25-hydroxyvitamin D and Safety, *Am J Clin Nutr*, 69, 1999, 842–856

Wharton, B. A., 'Low Plasma Vitamin D in Asian Toddlers in Britain', *British Medical Journal*, 18, 1999, 2–3

Wingo, P., et al., 'Cancer Incidence and Mortality 1973–1995', *Cancer*, March 15, 1998 1197–1207

Chapter 4

Annotations – 'Natural and Artificial Sun Cure in Tuberculosis of the Lungs', *Lancet*, 4th August 1923, 237–238.

Anon., 'A Smoking Gun? Drug Resistance in Hospitals has been traced to the Farmyard', *New Scientist*, 21 March 1998, 13

Anon., 'Theodore Kocher (1841–1917) Bernese Burgher', *J Am Med Assn*, April 17, 200, 3, 1967, 246–247

Anon., 'Obituary, Niels Ryberg Finsen, M.D.', *British Medical Journal* Oct. 1st, 1904, 865–866

Anon., House of Commons Environment Committee 7th Report, *'Indoor Air Pollution'*, HMSO, London, 1991

Anon., House of Lords, Science and Technology Committee 7th Report, 'Resistance to Antibiotics and other Antimicrobial Agents', The Stationery Office, London, 1998

Balsdon, J. P., *Life and Leisure in Ancient Rome*, The Bodley Head, London, 1969

Barker, A.E., 'An Address on a Useful Technique in Removing Tubercular Disease from the Hip Joint', *British Medical Journal*, January 19th, 1889, 121–123

Bernhard, O., *Light Treatment in Surgery*, Edward Arnold & Co., London, 1926

Bernhard, O. 'The Need for Climatic Sanatoria for Indigent Patients Suffering from Surgical Tuberculosis', *Journal of State Medicine*, 39, 6, June 1931, 333–345

Bodington, G. 'An Essay on the Treatment of Pulmonary Consumption, On Principles Natural, Rational and Successful', Longmans, 1840. Reprinted in *Selected Essays and Monographs*, The New Sydenham Society, London, MDCCCCI

Bryder, L., *Below the Magic Mountain – A Social History of Tuberculosis in Twentieth Century Britain*, Clarendon Press, Oxford, 1988

Carter A.J. 'Hugh Owen Thomas: the Cripples' Champion', *British Medical Journal*, Vol 303, 21–28, December 1991, 1578–1581

Cohen, M.L., 'Epidemiology of Drug Resistance: Implications for a Post–Antimicrobial Era', *Science*, 257, 21 August 1992, 1050–1054

Daniels, A., 'Why the Superbug isn't the End of the World', *The Sunday Telegraph*, 26th April 1998, 37

De Kruif, P., *Men Against Death*, Jonathan Cape, London, 1933

Dickinson, C.R., 'Niels R. Finsen – His Life and Work', *Transactions of the Canadian Institute*, V111, 1904–5, 99–135

Downes, A., and Blunt, T.P., 'Researches on the Effect of Light Upon Bacteria and Other Organisms', *Proc Roy Soc*, 26, 1877, 488–500

Dzielski, B., 'From Two Weeks to Twenty Two: One Patient's Experience of Minor Surgery', *J. Tissue Viability*, 9, 1, 1999, 17–19

Finsen, N.R. *Phototherapy*, Edward Arnold, London, 1901

Flachsmann, K., *Der Engadiner Arzt Oskar Bernhard (1861–1939) und die Begrundung der Heliotherapie bei der Chirurgischen Tuberkulose*, Schwabe & Company, Basel, 1966

Gauvain, H.J. 'Light Treatment in Surgical Tuberculosis', *Lancet*, April 19th 1927, 754–758

Harvard, C.W.H., (Ed.), *Black's Medical Dictionary*, 36th Edition, A. & C. Black, London, 1990

Hill, L.E., 'The Penetration of Rays through the Skin and Radiant Energy for the Treatment of Wounds', *Journal of the Royal Army Medical Corps*, LXXIV, 1, 1940, 1–9

Hippocrates, *Works of Hippocrates,* (Trans. and Eds. Jones, W.H.S. and Withington, E.T.), Harvard University Press Cambridge, Massachusetts, 1923–1931

Holubar, K., and Schmidt, C., 'Historical, Anthropological and Biological Aspects of Sun and the Skin', *Clinical Dermatology*, 16,1, 1998, 19–22

Houston, R.A., *Light and Colour,* London, Longmans, Green and Co., 1923

Jajic I., 'Balneotherapy and Heliomarinotherapy in the Treatment and Rehabilitation of Patients with Psoriatic Arthritis', *Reumatizam*, 31, 1–2, 1984, 13–6 (In Serbo–Croat)

Karimova, N.Kh., 'Concentrated Sunlight in the Therapy of Patients with Rheumatoid Arthritis', *Vopr Kurortol Fizioter Lech Fiz Kult* Sep–Oct, 5, 1988, 34–7 (In Russian)

Kobritsova, L.N., 'Climatotherapy', *Med Sestra,* 43, 5, 1984, 11–3 (In Russian)

Kocher, T., *Text Book of Operative Surgery,* (Trans. Stiles, H.J.) A. & C. Black, London, 1895

Krasik, Ia.D., Perelimuter, D.L., Liustin, V.N., and Kurganov, G.V., 'Changes in Hemodynamic Indices during Heliofangotherapy Procedures', *Vopr Kurortol Fizioter Lech Fiz Kult,* Jan–Feb, 1, 1984, 53–4 (In Russian)

Laurens, H., 'Sunlight and Health,' *Scientific Monthly,* 42, 1936, 312–324

Lilija, S., 'Sun-Bathing in Antiquity', *Arctos,* 21, 1987, 53–60

Lockhart Mummery, J. P., *Nothing New Under the Sun,* Andrew Melrose, London, 1947

Lomholt, S., 'Niels Ryberg Finsen 1860–1904' in *Prominent Danish Scientist through the Ages* (Ed. Meisen, V.) Levin and Munks Gaard Publishers, Copenhagen MCMXXXII

Lomholt, S. 'Die Forste Sollysbade for Tuberkulose – en Halvt Forglemt Episode', *Ugeskrift for Laeger,* Vol 92, September 25th, 1930, 915–916

Malikov, V.G., 'Method of traction treatment of pain syndromes', *Vrach Delo,* 9, Sept, 1983, 100–1 (In Russian)

Mayer, E., *Sunlight and Artificial Radiation,* Ballière, Tindall and Cox, London, 1926

Moffett, C., 'Dr Finsen and the Story of his Achievement', *McClure's Magazine,* February 1903, 361–368

Moynihan, B., 'An Address on the Treatment of Gunshot Wounds', *British Medical Journal*, March 4th, 1916, 333–339

Moynihan, G.S.E., *Lord Mayor Treloar Hospital and College,* Paul Cave Publications, Southampton, 1988

Obituary: 'Auguste Rollier, M.D.', *British Medical Journal*, November 13th, 1954, 1169–1170

Obituary: 'Auguste Rollier, M.D.', *British Medical Journal*, November 20th 1954, 1233

Obituary: 'Auguste Rollier', *Lancet*, November 13th, 1954, 1025

Pliny the Elder, *Natural History: A Selection,* (Trans. Healy J.F.) Penguin Books, London, 1991

Plowman, R. M., Graves, N. and Roberts, J. A., *Hospital Acquired Infection',* Office of Health Economics, London, 1997

Power, D., 'Sir Henry John Gauvain (1878–1945)', in *Lives of the Fellows of the Royal College of Surgeons of England,* London, 1953, 317–319

Rollier, A., *Le Pansement Solaire,* Payot & Co, Lausanne and Paris, 1916

Rollier, A., 'Tuberculosis Finds Cure in the Leysin Heliotherapy Clinics', *The Modern Hospital,* XXI, 3 September 1923, 255–260

Rollier, A., 'The Share of the Sun in the Prevention and Treatment of Tuberculosis', *British Medical Journal,* October 21st 1922, 741–745

Rollier, A., *Heliotherapy,* Oxford Medical Publications, London, Second Edition, 1927

Rollier, A., *Quarante Ans diHEliothErapie,* Lausanne, University of Lausanne, 1944

Rowbottom, R. and Susskind, C., *Electricity and Medicine: History of their Interaction,* San Francisco Press Inc, California, 1984

Sadykova, G.A., 'The Late Results of Helioaerotherapy in the Combined Treatment of Patients with Chronic Bronchitis', *Vopr Kurortol Fizioter Lech Fiz Kult,* Sep–Oct, 5, 1989, 57–8 (In Russian)

Saleeby, C.W., 'Sunlight and Disease', *Nature,* April 28th 1923, 574–576

Savorovskii, E.G., Danilova, M.I. and Kromer, V.V., 'A Solar Radiation Dosimeter for Heliotherapy', *Vopr Kurortol Fizioter Lech Fiz Kult,* 4, July–Aug., 1989, 65 (In Russian)

Scarborough, J., *Roman Medicine,* Thames and Hudson, London, 1969

Schrumpf–Pierron, B., 'Le Mal de Pott en Egypte 4000 Ans avant Notre Ere', *Aesculape,* 23, 1933, 295–299

Schuh, A., 'Climatotherapy,' *Experienta,* 49, 1993, 947–956

Sigerist, H.E., *A History of Medicine, Vol. I: Primitive and Archaic Medicine,* Oxford University Press, 1951

Sigerist, H.E., *Great Doctors,* Allen and Unwin, London, 2nd Edition, 1933

Scott, B.O., 'Clinical Uses of Ultraviolet Radiation', in Therapeutic Electricity and Ultraviolet Radiation, *Physical Medicine Library, Vol 4* (Ed. Licht, S.), Elizabeth Licht, New Haven, 1967

Smith F.B., *The Retreat of Tuberculosis* 1850–1950, Croom Helm, London, 1988

Snellman, E., Maljanen, T., et al., 'Effect of Heliotherapy on the Cost of Psoriasis', *British Journal of Dermatology,* 138, 2, 1998, 288–92

Stiles, H.J., 'Discussion on the After–Results of Major Operations for Tuberculosis Disease of the Joints', *British Medical Journal,* November 28th, 1912, 1356–1364

Waldram, P.J., Beckett, H.E., et al., *The Orientation of Buildings* – Being the Report of the RIBA Joint Committee on the Orientation of Buildings, Royal Institute of British Architects, London, 1933

Chapter 5

Anon., *The World Health Report,* World Health Organization, Geneva, 1997

Bishop, B., *A Time To Heal,* Penguin Arkana, London, 1996

Black, H.S., Thornby, J.I., Wolf, J.E. et al., 'Evidence that a Low–Fat Diet Reduces the Occurrence of Non–Melanoma Skin Cancer', *Int J Cancer,* 62, 1995, 165–169

Chamberlain, J., *Fighting Cancer,* Headline, London, 1997

Diffey B.L., 'Solar Radiation Effects on Biologic Systems', *Phys Med Biol,* 36, 1991 299–328

Downing, D., *Day Light Robbery,* Arrow Books, London, 1988

Erazmus, U., *Fats that Heal, Fats that Kill,* Alive Books, Burnaby, 1993

Gerber, M., 'Olive Oil, Monounsaturated Fatty Acids and Cancer', *Cancer Letters,* 1997 March, 114, 1–2, 91–2

Gerson, M., *A Cancer Treatment – Results of Fifty Cases,* 5th Edition, Gerson Institute, 1990

Goldberg, L.H., 'Basal Cell Carcinoma', *Lancet,* 9 March, 1996, 663–667

Hall, C., 'West is now Messenger of Death to Third World', *The Daily Telegraph,* 5 May, 1997, 6

Harris, A., *The Safe Tan Hand Book,* Sphere, 1989

Heaney, R. P., 'Lessons for Nutritional Science from Vitamin D', *Am J Clin Nutr,* 69, 825–826

Hildebrand, G.L., et al., 'Five Year Survival Rates of Melanoma Patients Treated by Diet Therapy after the Manner of Gerson', *Altern Ther Health Med,* 1 (14), 1995, 29–37

Holick, M.F., 'The Photobiology of Vitamin D and its Consequences for Humans', *Ann New York Acad Sci,* 453, 1985, 1–13

Holick M.F., 'Vitamin D and Bone Health', *J Nutr,* 126, 4, 1996 Suppl, 1159S–64S

Holick, M.F., 'Vitamin D – New Horizons for the 21st Century', *Am J Clin Nutrition,* 60, 1994, 619–630

Holick, M.F., 'Photosynthesis of Vitamin D in the Skin: Effect of Environment and Life–style Variables', *Fed Proc,* 46, 1987, 1876–1882

Kime, Z.R., *Sunlight Could Save Your Life,* World Health Publications, Penryn, California, 1980

Liberman, J.I., *Light: Medicine of the Future,* Bear & Co., Santa Fe, 1991

Lyttleton, J., 'Dietary Principles In Asian Folklore', *J Oriental Medicine*

MacLaughlin, J.A., Anderson, R.R., and Holick, M.F., 'Spectral Character of Sunlight Modulates Photosynthesis of Previtamin D3 and its Photoisomers in Human Skin', *Science,* 216, May 28, 1982, 4549, 1001–1003

Matsuoka, L. Y., Wortsman, J., et al., 'Clothing prevents Ultraviolet–B Radiation–dependent Photosynthesis of vitamin D3', *J. Clin Endocrine and Metab,* 75, 4, 1992, 1099–1092

Mo, T., and Green, A.E.S., 'A Climatology of Solar Erythema Dose', *Photochemistry and Photobiology,* Vol 20, 1974,483–496

Kemp, T., Pearce, N., Fitzharris, P., et al., 'Is Immunization a Risk Factor for Childhood Asthma or Allergy?', *Epidemiology,* 8, 6, Nov. 1997, 678–680

Kime, Z.R., *Sunlight Could Save Your Life,* World Health Publications, Penryn, California, 1980

Kohlmeier, L., 'Biomarkers of Fatty Acid and Breast Cancer Risk', *Am J Clin Nutr,* 66, 6, 1997 Suppl. 1548S–1556S

Kohlmeier, L., et al., 'Adipose Tissue Trans Fatty Acids and Breast Cancer', *Cancer Epidemiol Biomarkers Prevention,* 6, 9 1997, 705–710

Kuller, L.H. 'Dietary Fat and Chronic Diseases: Epidemiologic Overview', *J Am Diet Assoc,* 97, 7 1997, Suppl, S9–15

Leggett, D., *Helping Ourselves: A Guide to Traditional Chinese Food Energetics,* Meridian Press, Totnes, Devon, 1994

Shuttleworth, D., 'Sunbeds and the Pursuit of the Year Round Tan', *British Medical Journal,* 307, 11th December 1993, 1508–1509 1997, 1273–1278

Vieth, R., 'Vitamin D Supplementation, 25–Hydroxyvitamin D Concentrations, and Safety', *Am J Clin Nutr,* 69, 842–856

Weisburger, J.H., 'Dietary Fats and Risk of Chronic Disease: Mechanistic Insights from Experimental Studies', *J Am Diet Assoc,* 97, 1997 (suppl): S16–S23

Weitz, M., *Health Shock,* Hamlyn, Middlesex, 1982

Wellburn, A., *Air Pollution and Climate Change: The Biological Impact,* Longman, London, 1994

Chapter 6

Acra, A., Jurdi, M., MuiAllem, H., Karahagopian, Y. and Raffoul, Z., 'Sunlight as Disinfectant', *Lancet,* Feb 4, 1989, 280

Anon., 'Leaving the Comfort Zone', *M&E Design,* September 1997, 15–16

Anon., *Sick Building Syndrome: Causes, Effects and Controls,* London Hazards Centre, London, 1990

Atkinson, W., *The Orientation of Buildings or Planning for Sunlight,* Chapman and Hall, London, 1912

Barss, P., and Comfort, K., 'Ward Design and Jaundice in the Tropics: Report of an Epidemic', *British Medical Journal,* 291, 1985, 400–401

Beauchemin, K.M., and Hays, P., 'Dying in the Dark: Sunshine, Gender, and Outcomes in Myocardial Infarction', *J Roy Soc Medicine,* 91, July 1998, 352–354

Boubekri, M. 'Impact of Window Size and Sunlight Penetration on Office Workers' Mood and Satisfaction: a Novel Way of Assessing Sunlight', *Environment and Behaviour,* 4, July 23 1991, 474–493

Bristowe, J.S., and Holmes, T., *Report on Hospitals of the United Kingdom,* Sixth Report of the Medical Officer of the Privy Council, Appendix 15, HMSO, London, 1864, 463–762

Brundage, J.F., et al., 'Energy Efficient Buildings Pose Higher Risk of Respiratory Infection: Study', *J Am Med Assn,* 259, 14, 8 April 1988, 2108–2112

Buchbinder, L., 'The Bactericidal Effects of Daylight and Sunlight on Chained Gram Positive Cocci in Simulated Room Environment: Theoretical and Practical Considerations', in Aerobiology, (Ed. Moulton, F.R.), *American. Ass. Advancement of Science,* Smithsonian Institute, Washington, 1942, 267–270

Buchbinder, L., 'The Transmission of Certain Infections of Respiratory Origin', *J Am Med Assn,* Feb 28, 1942, 718–730

Burberry, P., *Environment and Services (Third edition),* Batsford, London, 1977

Burnett, J., *A Social History of Housing,* University Press, Cambridge, 1980

Butti, K., and Perlin, J., *A Golden Thread – 2500 Years of Solar Architecture and Technology,* Marion Boyars, London, 1980

Cowie, L.W., *A Dictionary of British Social History,* G. Bell and Sons Ltd., London, 1973

Dixon, R.E., 'Economic Costs of Respiratory Tract Infections in the United States', *Am J Med,* Vol 78 (Suppl 6B) 1985, 45–51

Douglas, C.G., 'Leonard Erskine Hill 1866–1952', *Obituary Notices of the Fellows of the Royal Society,* 22, November, 1953

Edmonds, R.L., (Ed.) *Aerobiology: The Ecological Systems Approach,* Dowden Hutchinson & Ross, Pennsylvania

Forty, A., *The Modern Hospital in England and France: the Social and Medical uses of Architecture in Buildings and Society,* (Ed. King, A.D.), Routledge and Keegan Paul, London, 1980, 61–93

Galton, D., *Healthy Hospitals,* Clarendon Press, Oxford, 1893

Garrod, L.P., 'Some Observations on Hospital Dust with Special Reference to Light as a Hygienic Safeguard', *British Medical Journal,* Feb 19, 1944, 245–257

Gauvain, H.J., 'Planning a Hospital', The Annual Oration, Transactions of the Medical Society of London, 61, May, 1938, 246–261

Gordon, R., *The Alarming History of Medicine,* Sinclair Stevenson, London, 1993

Hill, L.E., *Sunshine and Open-Air: Their Influence on Health with Special Reference to Alpine Climates (Second edition),* Edward Arnold and Co., London, 1925

Hill, L.E., and Argyll Campbell, J., 'Metabolism of Children Undergoing Open–Air Treatment', *British Medical Journal,* February 25th, 1922, 301–303

Hill, L.E., and Campell, A., *Health and Environment,* Edward Arnold and Co., London, 1925

Hollwich, F., *The Influence of Occular Light Perception on Metabolism on Man and in Animal,* Springer-Verlag, New York, 1979

Houk, V.N., Kent, D.C., et al., 'The Epidemiology of Tuberculosis Infection in a Closed Environment', *Arch Environ Health,* 16, 1968, 26–35

Hudson, B., and Hill, L., 'Some Clinical Observations on Heliotherapy in Pulmonary Tuberculosis', *Lancet,* June 7th 1924, 1147

Jewess, B.W., 'Some Medical Uses of Radiation from Lamps', *Lighting Research and Technology,* 10, 4, 1978, 184–188

Johnson, B.G., Kronvall, J., Lindvall, et al., *Buildings and Health – Indoor Climate and Effective Energy Use,* Swedish Council for Building Research, Stockholm, Sweden, 1991

Kenyon, T.A., Valway, S.E., Ihle, W.W., Onorato, I.M. and Castro, K.G., 'Transmission of Multi–Drug Resistant Mycobacterium Tuberculosis during a Long Plane Flight', *N Eng J Med,* 334, 15, 1996, 933–938

King, A., 'Hospital Planning: Revised Thoughts on the Origin of the Pavilion Principle in England', *Medical History,* 10, 1966, 360–373

'Levy, S.B., 'The Challenge of Antibiotic Resistance', *Scientific American,* March 1998, 32–39

Liberman, J.I., *Light: Medicine of the Future,* Bear & Co., Santa Fe, 1991

LLoyd Wright, F., *The Natural House,* Horizon Press 1954 (Reprint: Pitman, London, 1971)

Milton, R., *Forbidden Science,* Fourth Estate, London, 1994

Murray, I., 'Hospital Infections Kill More Than Road Crashes', *The Times,* September 16th 1997, 6

Neieman, E., Light, W. and Hopkinson, R.G., 'Recommendations for the Admission and Control of Sunlight in Buildings', *Building and Environment,* 11, 1976, 91–101

Nightingale, F., *Notes on Hospitals (Third edition),* Longman, Roberts and Green, London, 1863

Obituary, 'Leonard Erskine Hill', *Lancet,* April 12th, 1952, 771–772

Obituary, 'Sir Leonard Hill', *British Medical Journal,* April 5th, 1952, 767–768

Page, J.K. (Ed.), *Indoor Environment: Health Aspects of Air Quality, Thermal Environment, Light and Noise,* WHO/EHE/RUD/90.2, World Health Organization, Geneva, 1990

Pearson, D., *The Natural House Book,* Simon and Schuster, New York, 1989

Ransome, A., and Delephine, S., 'On the Influence of Natural Agents on the Virulence of the Tubercle Bacillus', *Proc Roy Soc of London,* 1894, Vol 56, 51–56.

Ransome, A., *The Principles of 'Open-Air' Treatment of Phthisis and of Sanatorium Construction,* London, Smith Elder & Co., 1903

Redlich, C.A., and Cullen, M.R., 'Sick Building Syndrome,' *Lancet,* 349, 5 April, 1997, 1013–1016

Reid, I.R., Gallagher, D.J. and Bogsworth, J., 'Prophylaxis Against Vitamin D Deficiency in the Elderly by Regular Sunlight Exposure', *Age and Ageing*, 15, 1986, 35–40

Simon, J., 'Hospital Statistics and Hospital Hygiene', Sixth Report of the Medical Officer of the Privy Council, Part II, 4, HMSO, London, 1864, 37–74

Small, H., *Florence Nightingale Avenging Angel*, Constable, London, 1998

Taylor, J.R.B., *Hospital and Asylum Architecture in England 1840–1914*, Mansell, 1990

Thorington, L., 'Spectral, Irradiance and Temporal Aspects of Natural Light', *Ann New York Acad Sci*, 453, 1985, 5421–5427

Venolia, C., 'Health, Buildings and the Sun', *SunWorld*, 12, 2, 1988, 48–51

Vitruvius, *The Ten Books on Architecture*, (Trans. Hickey Morgan, M.,) Dover, New York, 1960

Waldram, P.J., and Beckett, H.E., *The Orientation of Buildings* – Being the Report of the RIBA Joint Committee on the Orientation of Buildings, Royal Institute of British Architects, London, 1933

Wilson, R., 'Something in the Air', Scottish Television Enterprises for Dispatches, Channel 4 Television, London, January 1998

Woodham–Smith, C., *Florence Nightingale 1820–1910*, Fontana, London, 1977

Yannas, S., *Solar Energy and Housing Design, Volume 1*, Architectural Association, London, 1994

Chapter 7

Anon., *The World Health Report*, World Health Organization, Geneva, 1997

Brecher, P., *Principles of Tai Chi*, Thorsons, London, 1997

Chang, S.T., and Miller, C., *Burn Disease Out of Your Body*, Thorsons Publishers, Northampton, 1984

Cho, T.H., *Knocking at the Gate of Life and other Healing Exercises from China: The Official Exercise Book of the People's Republic of China*, (Trans. Chang, E.), Rodale Press, Emmaus, PA, USA, 1985

Garland, F.C, and Garland, C.F., 'Occupational Sunlight Exposure and Melanoma in the U.S. Navy', *Archives of Environmental Health*, 45, 5, 1990, 261–267

Gauvain, H.J., 'Reflections on Sun Treatment: The Theory of Varying Stimuli and Varying Response', *The Practitioner*, CXXXII, February, 1934, 156–165

Kevan, S.M., 'Quest for Cures: a History of Tourism for Climate and Health', *Int J Biometeriol*, 37, 1993, 113–124

Kaptchuck, T.J., *Chinese Medicine: The Web That Has No Weaver*, Rider & Co., London, 1989

Kit, W.K., *The Art of Chi Kung*, Element Books, London, 1993

Kit, W.K., *The Complete Book of Tai Chi Chuan*, Element Books, London, 1997

Kenyon, J., *21st Century Medicine*, Thorsons, Northampton, 1986

Kutner, N.G., Barnhart, H., Wolf, S.L., 'Self–Report Benefits of Tai Chi Practice by Older Adults', *J Gerontol*, Series B, 52, 5, September 1996, 242

Maciocia, G., *The Foundations of Chinese Medicine*, Churchill Livingstone, London, 1989

Needham, J., 'Science and Civilisation in China', Volume 2, *History of Scientific Thought*, Cambridge University Press, 1956

Nieves, J., Cosman, F., Herbert J., et al., 'High Prevalence of Vitamin D Deficiency and Reduced Bone Mass in MS', *Neurology*, 44, 9, 1687–1692

Randle, H.W., 'Suntanning: Differences in Perceptions Throughout History', *Mayo Clin Proc*, 72, 5, 1997, 461–6

Sato, Y., Kikuyama, M., and Oizumi, K., 'High Prevalence of Vitamin D Deficiency and Reduced Bone Mass In Parkinson's Disease', *Neurology*, 49, 5

Schwartzman, L., 'Tai Chi is Helpful to Parkinson's Patients', *Tai Chi*, 22,1, February 1998, 32–33

Tse, M., *Qigong for Health and Vitality*, Piatkus, 1997

Wolf, S.L., Coogler, C., and Xu, T., 'Exploring the Basis for Tai Chi Chuan as a Therapeutic Exercise Approach', *Arch Phys Med Rehab*, 78, August 1997, 886–892

RECOMMENDED READING

Arnold, A., *Winners*, Paladin, London, 1989

Butti, K., and Perlin, J., *A Golden Thread*, Marion Boyars, London, 1980

Bishop, B., *A Time To Heal*, Penguin Arkana, London, 1996

Chaitow, L., *Vaccination and Immunisation: Dangers, Delusions and Alternatives*, C.W. Daniel Company Ltd., Saffron Walden, 1994

Chamberlain, J., *Fighting Cancer*, Headline, London, 1997

Coleman, V., *Bodypower*, European Medical Journals, Barnstaple, Devon, 1994

Downing, D., *Day Light Robbery*, Arrow Books, London, 1988

Erazmus, U., *Fats that Heal, Fats that Kill*, Alive Books, Burnaby, 1993

Gordon, R., *The Alarming History of Medicine*, Sinclair–Stevenson, London, 1993

Gerson, M., *A Cancer Treatment – Results of Fifty Cases*, 5th Edition, Gerson Institute, 1990

Illich, I., *Medical Nemesis – the Limits to Medicine*, Penguin, London, 1975

Kime, Z.R., *Sunlight Could Save Your Life*, World Health Publications, Penryn, California, 1980

Liberman, J.I., *Light: Medicine of the Future*, Bear & Co., Santa Fe, 1991

Marsh, E., *Black Patent Shoes: Dancing with MS*, Sideroad Press, Ontario, 1996

McTaggart, L., *What Doctors Don't Tell You*, Thorsons, London, 1996

Milton, R., *Forbidden Science*, Fourth Estate, London, 1994

Ott, J.N., *Health and Light*, Pocket Books, New York, 1973

Rosenthal, N., *Winter Blues*, Fontana, 1991

Rowe, D., *Breaking the Bonds*, Fontana, London, 1991

Shaw, B., *The Doctor's Dilemma*, Penguin, London, 1979

Smyth, A., *Seasonal Affective Disorder*, Thorsons, London, 1995

Small, H., *Florence Nightingale Avenging Angel*, Constable, London, 1998

Weitz, M., *Health Shock*, Hamlyn, Middlesex, 1982

INDEX

K

L

M

N

O

P

tuberculosis   13, 16, 17, 53, 63, 67, 76,
       85, 87, 91, 94, 98, 99, 102, 103,
       106, 110, 128, 132, 133, 149, 151
Tutenkamun   30

U

UK Department of Health   20, 26
UK Skin Cancer Prevention
   Working Party   26
ultraviolet A (UVA)   18, 23, 35, 48, 127
ultraviolet B (UVB)   18, 23, 24, 35, 48,
                              114, 117, 127
ultraviolet radiation   17, 19, 22, 24, 27, 42,
       47, 50, 61, 79, 92, 94, 111, 117,
       118, 119, 122, 127, 128
United States   21, 23, 58, 60
University of Vienna's Institute of
   Human Biology   28
US Navy   47
USS Richard E Byrd   133

V

varicose ulcers   107
VDUs   144
ventilation   135, 137, 139, 146
vernal equinox   116

viral infections   85
vitamin D   14, 18, 22, 24, 26, 29, 38,
       40, 49, 55, 58, 60, 62, 66, 69, 78,
       79, 111, 113, 114, 147, 150, 154, 155
vitamin D deficiency   20, 36, 56, 61, 63,
                           69, 113, 128, 150
vitamin D insufficiency 20, 58, 78, 148, 150
Vitamin D Winter   18
vitamins   15, 19, 20, 51, 58, 119, 124
Vitruvius   130, 133, 141, 157

W

Walter, Dr Otto   89
war wounds   15, 53, 95, 98, 149
Ward, Sister   28
Widmark, Professor Erik Johan   92
Window Tax   131
winter solstice   115
World Health Organization   34, 60, 78, 151
wounds   96, 99, 110

Z

zeitgebers   17, 19, 32
Zhang San Feng   153
zymotic theory   138, 139

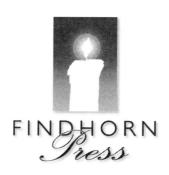

FINDHORN Press

Findhorn Press is the publishing business of the Findhorn Community which has grown around the Findhorn Foundation in northern Scotland.

For further information about the Findhorn Foundation and the Findhorn Community, please contact:

Findhorn Foundation

The Visitors Centre
The Park, Findhorn IV36 3TY, Scotland, UK
tel 01309 690311• fax 01309 691301
email reception@findhorn.org
www.findhorn.org

For a complete Findhorn Press catalogue, please contact:

Findhorn Press

The Park, Findhorn,
Forres IV36 3TY
Scotland, UK
Tel 01309 690582
freephone 0800-389 9395
Fax 01309 690036

P. O. Box 13939
Tallahassee
Florida 32317-3939, USA
Tel (850) 893 2920
toll-free 1-877-390-4425
Fax (850) 893 3442

e-mail info@findhornpress.com
findhornpress.com